Health and Industrial Growth

The Ciba Foundation for the promotion of international cooperation in
medical and chemical research is a scientific and educational charity established by
CIBA Limited – now CIBA-GEIGY Limited – of Basle. The Foundation operates
independently in London under English trust law.

Ciba Foundation Symposia are published in collaboration with
Associated Scientific Publishers (Elsevier Scientific Publishing Company, Excerpta Medica,
North-Holland Publishing Company) in Amsterdam.

Associated Scientific Publishers, P.O. Box 211, Amsterdam

Health and Industrial Growth

Ciba Foundation Symposium 32 (new series)

1975

Elsevier · Excerpta Medica · North-Holland

Associated Scientific Publishers · Amsterdam · Oxford · New York

© *Copyright 1975 Ciba Foundation*

Science
RA
565
A1
S95
1974

ISBN Excerpta Medica 90 219 4036 1
ISBN American Elsevier 0-444-15180-x

Published in August 1975 by Associated Scientific Publishers, P.O. Box 211, Amsterdam and American Elsevier, 52 Vanderbilt Avenue, New York, N.Y. 10017.

Suggested series entry for library catalogues: Ciba Foundation Symposia.
Suggested publisher's entry for library catalogues: Associated Scientific Publishers.

Ciba Foundation Symposium 32 (new series)

Printed in The Netherlands by Van Gorcum, Assen

Contents

Participants

Symposium on Health and Industrial Growth, held at the Ciba Foundation, London, 11th–13th September 1974

Chairman: LORD ASHBY The Master's Lodge, Clare College, Cambridge CB2 1TL

M. BAVANDI Division of Health & Social Welfare, Plan and Budget Organization, PO Box 12–1244, Tehran, Iran

H. BRIDGER The Tavistock Institute of Human Relations, The Tavistock Centre, 120 Belsize Lane, London NW3 5BA

E. J. CHALLIS Petrochemicals Division, Imperial Chemical Industries Ltd., P.O. Box 90, Wilton, Middlesbrough, Cleveland County TS6 8JE

L. K. A. DERBAN Volta River Authority, P.O. Box M77, Accra, Ghana

H. DICKINSON School of Engineering Science, University of Edinburgh, King's Buildings, Mayfield Road, Edinburgh EH9 3JL

M. A. EL BATAWI Occupational Health Unit, World Health Organization, 1211 Geneva 27, Switzerland

J. C. GILSON MRC Pneumoconiosis Unit, Llandough Hospital, Penarth, Glamorgan CF6 1XW

W. W. HOLLAND Department of Clinical Epidemiology and Social Medicine, St Thomas's Hospital Medical School, Albert Embankment, London SE1 7EH

I. ILLICH Center for Intercultural Documentation (CIDOC), Apartado 479, Cuernavaca, Mexico, CA

W. T. JONES District Community Physician, Harrow and Brent Area Health Authority, District Offices, Central Middlesex Hospital, Park Royal, London N.W.10

N. Y. KIROV   Department of Fuel Technology, School of Chemical Engineering, The University of New South Wales, P.O. Box 1, Kensington, N.S.W., Australia 2033

W. L. KISSICK   Department of Community Medicine, University of Pennsylvania, Philadelphia, USA

P. J. LAWTHER   MRC Air Pollution Unit, St Bartholomew's Hospital Medical College, Charterhouse Square, London EC1M 6BQ

G. MARS   The Tavistock Institute of Human Relations (CDIC), The Tavistock Centre, 120 Belsize Lane, London NW3 5BA

R. MURRAY   Burchetts, Newton Green, Sudbury, Suffolk CO10 OQZ

V. PAPANEK   School of Industrial Design, Carleton University, Colonel By Drive, Ottawa, Canada

J. R. PHILIP   Division of Environmental Mechanics, CSIRO, P.O. Box 821, Canberra City, A.C.T., Australia 2601

W. O. PHOON   Department of Social Medicine and Public Health, University of Singapore, Outram Hill, Singapore 3

R. S. PORTER   Economic Planning, Ministry of Overseas Development, Eland House, Stag Place, London SW1E 5DH

V. RAMALINGASWAMI   All India Institute of Medical Sciences, Ansari Nagar, New Delhi–16, India

H. SAKABE   National Institute of Industrial Health, Ministry of Labour, 2051 Kizukisumiyoshi-Cho, Kawasaki, Japan

A. WHITE   Institute of Development Studies, Sussex University, Falmer, Brighton BN1 9QH

J. C. WOOD   Department of Law, Sheffield University, Sheffield S10 2TN

Editors: KATHERINE ELLIOTT *(Organizer)* and JULIE KNIGHT

Preface

Just over two years ago Lord Ashby suggested that the Ciba Foundation might usefully hold a discussion on second-order effects of industrial growth in relation to human health. The United Kingdom underwent industrialization in the late 18th and early 19th centuries. Other western countries soon followed suit. If appropriate experts, drawn from areas at various stages of industrialization, looked together at the UK experience, could some practical guidelines for development planners, politicians and legislators emerge?

It so happened that the symposium planning period coincided with dramatic world changes. These shifts sharpened the need to question our assumptions about the inevitable and beneficial nature of industrial development. We had set out to consider how possible ill-effects of industrialization on health could be either avoided or neutralized, but much more profound questions became unavoidably central to the symposium theme. Does the process of industrializing genuinely enhance the sum total of human well-being? Or may the changes involved so distort and harm a society that increasing prosperity fails to benefit those least able to fend for themselves?

This book, which records the papers and the discussions at the symposium held in 1974, begins with the more specific (although large and challenging enough) problems of the directly harmful side-effects of industrial growth. The ways in which control of pollution in the UK is approached are analysed, together with the contribution legislation can make to the protection of health at work. The symposium then widens out to consider the industrial 'growing pains' of developing countries and how they might avoid repeating mistakes made in 19th-century Europe. The impact of industrialization on health is taken up from viewpoints varying from Ghana, Iran and India to the South-East Asian region and Japan. The health of the working population in these countries is specifically examined, together with the question of how health

1

needs and problems of the workers can be integrated with those of the whole population, of which the workers are also a part.

In the final sections even wider, and probably generally relevant, problems of the impact of industrialized society as such on mankind's health and well-being are considered. The individual cannot be thought of separately from his or her family, work and environment; there has to be a holistic approach consistent with the social system accepted by a nation. The book takes us beyond the simpler issues of occupational hazards and effects of environmental pollutants to discuss concepts of health, disease and medical care in a rapidly changing world where universally rising hopes, demands and needs have somehow to be matched with finite and unequally distributed resources.

KATHERINE ELLIOTT

Legislation outside the factory: the British philosophy of pollution control

ERIC ASHBY

Some people may regard it as an abuse of the word 'philosophy' to use it in the context of pollution control. But I can defend the use of the word, for one of its approved meanings is 'the general principles of some particular activity'. That is what this paper is about.

The history of pollution control in Britain can be summarized as a succession of chain-reactions. Some nuisance in the environment, which people may have tolerated for years (a fog, the stink from a river, the noise of traffic) reaches an intolerable level and generates protest from the public. The protest is fanned into flame (e.g. by the mass media, pressure groups, and questions in Parliament). The government are obliged to take note of it. They may play for time by appointing a committee to enquire into the nuisance. The committee comes up with recommendations which are based on a rational appraisal of the situation. But rational appraisal is only one ingredient in the political decision which may follow. It now has to be decided whether the recommendations are politically viable. If they are, steps are taken to abate the nuisance. Action may take the form of new laws, or regulations, or a voluntary agreement on the part of the polluters to abate their pollution.

This is the typical succession of events. But conditioning each step in the succession there are social norms based on values; it is these which influence political decisions, and which constitute the 'philosophy' of pollution control.

First, consider the event which triggers off the chain-reaction leading to the control of pollution. The common cause is disquiet about health. In the 1850's outbreaks of cholera in London provoked the first serious steps to control river pollution in the Thames. In the 1950's some 4000 deaths attributed to the smog in December 1952 provoked the Clean Air Acts. The response to environmental health hazards is contagious. When 33 persons in Japan, over some 6–8 years in the 1950's, died after eating fish containing mercury, other coun-

3

tries round the world were alerted to the danger of releasing mercury into the sea. In 1970 high levels of methylmercury were found in some canned tuna fish, whereupon the British Government announced a scheme for the monitoring of foodstuffs for mercury and other heavy metals in this country, and set up a working party which published analyses of mercury in fish caught in the coastal waters of England and Wales[1]. Its conclusion was that the levels found were not high enough to endanger health, and there has been no legislative response to the discovery.

But proved danger to health is by no means the sole starting point for a chain-reaction to control pollution. It is commonly assumed, for instance, that visible and untreated domestic sewage in the sea and the presence in the atmosphere of carbon monoxide and lead from motor vehicles in Britain are dangerous to health; but the bulk of medical evidence does not support these assumptions. Nevertheless public opinion, fortified by pressure groups concerned for the environment, is prevailing against the resistance of other interests and is obliging governments to diminish these kinds of pollution at considerable public cost. The motive of governments in complying with these pressures could be regarded as a manifestation of prudence, on the ground that no-one knows what the long-term effects of low levels of pollution may be; however, it is more likely to be a non-rational, but nonetheless important, response to rising social norms, themselves the consequence of rising social values. For years the British people accepted fogs and stinking rivers and unsightly waste dumps, just as they accepted homes without indoor plumbing. Today conditions like these are regarded as an affront to public taste. Governments are therefore obliged to legislate against them even though there is no convincing evidence that they are a menace to public health. Clean air, rivers which can support fish, and waste dumps which are hidden from view are now considered to be desirable amenities, for which the public are prepared to instruct their legislators to pay. Therefore, in discussions of health and the environment, the word 'health' has to be extended in two ways: one, to cover the health not only of people, but of the biological cycles in rivers and estuaries, and the purity of the atmosphere; and the other, to cover, in human health, not only clinical disorders but the effects of the environment on stress, *anomie;* on what is described, but cannot be defined, as quality of life. And similar extensions of the word 'health' are relevant to discussions on health and industrial growth.

The second stage of the chain-reaction for pollution control is the building up of a sufficient pressure of opinion to alert administrators or governments to the need for action. This is the task for pressure groups, conservation lobbies, and individual enthusiasts. Almost invariably they lay themselves open to the charge of being 'unsound' because they adulterate rational argument with histrionic advocacy. But one has an uncomfortable feeling that, distasteful as it is to scientists, this is a necessary attribute at this stage of the process. For instance, four years ago there was published an impressive report of the Study of Critical Environmental Problems[2]. It was welcomed by experts; but it had no popular appeal until a garbled and sensational version of it appeared two years later as *A Blueprint for Survival*[3]. The response to this version was so lively that the Secretary of State deemed it prudent to give an interview to some of the signatories to it. One is reminded of Cardinal Newman's aphorism: 'Deductions have no power of persuasion...Many a man will live and die upon a dogma: no man will be a martyr for a conclusion'.[4]

The third common stage in the chain-reaction is the appointment of a committee of enquiry by Parliament or by a minister or (for issues of greater importance) the appointment of a royal commission. The facts are examined and assessed with clinical detachment. Experts of various kinds are called as witnesses. Any emotional and political overgrowth which may have confused the issue at the second stage is stripped away. The findings are published, often as parliamentary papers. These official reports constitute the basic evidence on which political or administrative decisions are made. Thus it was the report[5] of a select committee under Lord Derby in 1862 which led to the creation of the Alkali Inspectorate in England in 1863; a committee of the Ministry of Housing and Local Government under Sir Hugh Beaver (1954)[6] which led to the Clean Air Acts; and reports of the Royal Commission on Environmental Pollution (1971–1973) which preceded the composite Control of Pollution Act of 1974. But even these documents cannot be regarded as objective and disinterested analyses of the facts alone; they, too, reflect the social values of those who signed them. If their recommendations are to be taken seriously they can aim no higher, and must aim no lower, than the norms of reasonable and enlightened citizens at the time.

Finally, the issue comes on to the desk of the administrator and the politician. It is at this point that the characteristic British policy for dealing with environmental problems becomes manifest. There is, broadly, a choice between two models for controlling pollution. One model is to set standards for the *quality* of air or water which it is in the public interest to achieve, and to compel those who discharge wastes into the environment to limit their discharge so that these standards are maintained, regardless of cost or of possible second-order effects, such as the creation of unemployment in firms which cannot afford to comply with the standards. This model requires constant monitoring of the environment and procedures, often in courts of law, against polluters who overload it. The alternative model is to issue permits to discharge wastes into the environment, under conditions negotiated separately with each polluter. The polluter is required to strike a balance between the benefit to his industry (and hence to society) of the right to put his wastes into the environment and the benefits society will derive from cleaner air or water. The principle is that the polluter is not required to minimize his pollution; he is required to optimize it.

This second model is the one adopted in Britain. We do not, as some other countries do, set air quality standards covering an entire region. We require polluters to use what the statute describes as 'the best practicable means' for abating pollution. Thus the standard of abatement required for emissions of sulphur dioxide from a newly built factory may be much more severe than that required for an obsolete factory half a mile away, which has only a limited life. Similarly the demand for treatment of effluent into a river may be less severe downstream than upstream, and less for a lame industry, which might go out of business if put to great expense, than for a prosperous industry. The law for water is that discharges into rivers, estuaries, and the sea, require the consent of an authority (in this case the Regional Water Authority), but the terms for each individual consent are at the discretion of the Inspectorate and are not laid down by law. The year 1974 is the centennial of the formula 'the best practicable means'. The first legislation to deal with noxious vapours, in 1863, was restricted to the control of emissions of hydrochloric acid, and it did prescribe an emission standard, namely that 95% of the acid should be removed. But the apparently vaguer criterion of 'the best practicable means' was introduced because, as the Chief Alkali Inspector wrote in his report for 1887, it 'would prove an elastic band ever tightening as chemical science advanced and placed greater facilities in the hands of the manufacturer'.

This pragmatic system may seem open to criticism as untidy, indecisive and liable to abuse. If it were not administered by persons of high integrity and a strong sense of duty, there might be grounds for these criticisms. But in fact the system works. There are, of course, lapses and mistakes and they get pitiless publicity; the successes are not news.

There is, however, one justified criticism, which clauses in the Control of Pollution Act 1974 should remove. It is criticism against the confidentiality which has hitherto shielded the decisions of consenting authorities from public scrutiny. The 'deal' agreed between an alkali inspector and a ceramic works, or between a water authority and a pharmaceutical firm, allowing waste to be discharged into air or water, is not disclosed. The reason—not a convincing one—is that disclosure might give away trade secrets. This confidentiality generates suspicion—much of it unjustified—of the independence of the authority. The new legislation will do away with this; it will oblige authorities to keep registers of consents, to which the public shall have access.

How is the British 'philosophy' for pollution control operated? There are three practicable procedures, two of them already in common use; the third has been much discussed but not yet introduced. I shall give examples of each procedure.

The first is voluntary agreement among manufacturers to replace a polluting substance by a non-pollutant. An example of this is the elimination of non-biodegradable anionic surface-active ingredients from detergents. By 1956 Britain was using over 40 000 tons a year of a branched alkyl benzene sulphonate in domestic detergents. The substance was found to have serious second-order effects. It interfered with the treatment of sewage; it contaminated rivers with billows of foam; as little as 0.1 parts per million in rivers interfered with oxygen uptake; it was poisonous to some fish and water plants. The press took up the issue; photographs of 'detergent swans' were published; questions were asked in Parliament. In 1957 a Standing Technical Committee on Synthetic Detergents was set up. The very existence of the committee prompted the manufacturers to seek alternative anionic surface-active ingredients. By 1959 an unbranched alkyl benzene sulphonate, which was biodegradable and therefore had no objectionable second-order effects (a so-called 'soft' detergent), was given trials in two towns whose sewage discharged into the River Lee (see the Third Report of the Standing Technical Committee on Synthetic Detergents, 1960[8]). By 1964 the committee secured a voluntary undertaking by the manufacturers not to market 'hard' detergents for domestic use and by 1971 some 95 % of detergents on the market were 'soft'. The pollution was controlled at, as it were, the third stage of the chain-reaction of events without any action on the part of government at all. Similar undertakings have brought about dramatic reductions in the discharge into the environment of certain organochlorine compounds.

The abatement of smoke in Britain (a reduction from some 2.31 million tons in 1953 to about 0.7 million tons in 1974) is due partly to the replacement of coal by natural gas; but it is due, too, to voluntary action at the level of local government. The Clean Air Acts do not prescribe one blanket air quality standard for British cities; they leave the initiative to local authorities to designate areas under the Acts, whereupon it becomes obligatory to use smokeless fuels in these areas. Accordingly there are industrial cities, like Sheffield, where the Clean Air Acts have been introduced, and non-industrial towns where they have not.

The second procedure for the abatement of pollution is by legislation. This legislation (for example, the comprehensive Control of Pollution Act, which received the royal assent in 1974) illustrates clearly the British 'philosophy'. Nothing in the Act or in previous legislation *prohibits* the discharge of wastes into air, water, or land; nor does it anywhere prescribe air or water quality

TABLE 1

Examples of the abatement of pollution achieved by modernized methods of manufacture

Process	Pollution	Pollution as kilograms per tonne of product	
Nitric acid	Acid gases	Old	20
		New	7
Sulphuric acid	Acid gases	Old	6.7
		New	2.5
Terephthalic acid	BOD[a]	Old	13
		New	1.5
Ethylene	BOD	Old	1.3
		New	0.2
Ammonia	BOD	Old	3.8
		New	0.3

Source: Data from the Third Report[7] of the Royal Commission on Environmental Pollution (1972), p. 26.
[a] BOD, biological oxygen demand.

standards. What the Act does is to prohibit discharges *without the consent* of the appropriate authority. It is left to the authority to decide, for each individual polluter, where he should dump his toxic waste, or at what chimney-height he may discharge sulphur dioxide into the air, or in what concentrations he may release chemicals into sewers.

This pragmatic procedure must be judged by its results. Although the total emission of sulphur dioxide in the UK from 1958 to 1968 increased from about 5.8 to about 6 million tons, the average ground-level concentrations decreased from about 175 to about 110 micrograms per cubic metre (see the First Report of the Royal Commission on Environmental Pollution[7]). And industrial discharges into rivers—though still objectionably high—were steadily improved under pressure from the consent authorities. This improvement is evident from the figures for pollution (expressed as acid gases or biological oxygen demand, BOD) per tonne of product produced in old and new plant. Some examples are given in Table 1.

Attached to both these procedures—those entered upon voluntarily and those permitted under legislation—there is the popular declaration: 'the polluter must pay for his pollution'. This declaration needs to be examined, for it is liable to misinterpretation. It does not mean that the polluter pays for the damage done by his pollution; and this is just as well, for there are no trustworthy ways to assess the damage, even the damage to health. It does mean that the polluter has to comply with the terms or the consent or the licence under which he is permitted to put wastes into the environment. To this extent he internalizes some but not all of the social costs of his activity, and, of course, passes them on to the consumer.

The third practicable procedure for abating pollution is not yet fully introduced, but it is consistent with the British 'philosophy' and there is provision for it in Clause 45 of the Control of Pollution Act. It is to 'sell' the right to discharge wastes into the environment, on the principle that the environment is a limited resource under government surveillance. It is important to distinguish two kinds of charges. One is simply payment by the polluter to another body (such as a sewage works) for purifying his effluent before it reaches the river; that might be cheaper for the polluter than being obliged to set up his own sewage plant. The other kind of charge is one which would be levied by the authority responsible for the environment (e.g. the Regional Water Authority for a river; the Local Authority for smoke into the air). Its purpose would not be to pay for damage done, nor would it be levied in order to bring in revenue. It would be a device to persuade polluters to abate their pollution. Its level would be related to three parameters: (a) the amount of competition to put wastes into the local environment (e.g. in a city, the air above it and the river running through it); (b) the capacity of the environment to dispose of wastes (this would depend on the site of the city and the volume of water-flow in the river); and (c) the quality of environment which the local community wants (a value judgement which would have to strike a balance between the amenity value of clean air and water and the costs of achieving these, for example in the rates—local taxes—or in the effects on employment).

These three parameters vary greatly from place to place. The opinion of Lord Justice Thesiger, given in court nearly 100 years ago, is still valid law: that 'what would be a nuisance in Belgrave Square would not necessarily be so in Bermondsey'[9]. That is why a flexible system of charging polluters for the right to put wastes into the environment (with notionally 'cheap' and 'expensive' zones of air and water) would be a more efficient way to control pollution than to establish air and water quality standards, monitor them, and restrain those who offend against them.

The purpose of these reflections on the 'philosophy' of pollution control in Britain is to raise questions which are relevant to the theme of this symposium. Here are three such questions:

(1) Does one always have to wait for a publicized crisis before the mechanisms for preventing future crises are put into gear? Put in more general terms: are there ways in which a community can be persuaded to adapt its social values in anticipation of, rather than in response to, changes due to industrial growth? Past experience is not reassuring. Not only in pollution, but in other episodes,

it has needed a crisis before governments act. Examples are the control of antibiotics in animal feedstuffs, and the setting up of the Committee on the Safety of Drugs after the thalidomide tragedy.

(2) However, it is surely not necessary for nations in, as it were, an adolescent stage of technological growth to have to recapitulate in their ontogeny the whole drab phylogeny of industrial history. It is important that developing countries should enjoy the material benefits of the most up-to-date technology. But is it not just as important that the social norms of the citizens of developing countries should be higher than our social norms were a century or less ago, when our ancestors put up with environmental conditions which we would reject with horror? 'The pestilential smell from the Thames is becoming intolerable', wrote the Earl of Malmesbury in his diary (1884) 'and there has been a question of changing the locality of Parliament. Nothing can be done during this heat'.[10] It was not only the stink: tens of thousands died of cholera in London alone due to the primitive sanitary conditions. The air was no better than the water. Evidence given to Lord Derby's committee in 1862 spoke of 'certain districts of England absolutely desolated, as far as vegetation is concerned, by the works of man. Whole tracts of country, once as fertile as the fields of Devonshire, have been swept by deadly blights till they are as barren as the shores of the Dead Sea...' That was what the chemical industry was allowed to do only a little over a century ago. It was avoidable then—the technology for condensing the acid vapours existed—but the will to avoid it was absent. Can the developing countries mobilize the public opinion of their citizens, in their legitimate struggle for higher material standards of living, to ensure that this struggle does not endanger the health of man or his environment?

(3) And this leads to the third question. The recent history of pollution control demonstrates that social norms as to what is an acceptable environment are rising all the time, and that there is public consent for massive expenditure on pollution control even though there is no clear evidence that pollution is affecting health (as ordinarily understood). Therefore, in considering health and industrial growth, should one adopt a very broad concept of health, to mean much more than freedom from clinical disorders? Should low noise levels, easily accessible recreational facilities, absence of stress in travel to work, and stretches of pleasant landscape, be regarded as conducive to good mental health, and therefore be included in planning policies for industrial growth?

Discussion

White: It is an implicit assumption in your paper that the underdeveloped countries face the same problems we faced and are going through the same sort of process that we, in the industrialized countries, underwent 100 years ago; are therefore meeting the same problems; and so can benefit from our advice about our mistakes and from following our solutions. To my mind, this view is basically mistaken. Developing countries are not simply at an earlier stage of the same process but in a different process—a process which differs precisely because of the changes made to the world by our industrialization. Through our own industrialization we have developed highly capital-intensive machinery which is being imported by today's underdeveloped countries. These imports leave no opportunities, or far too few, for *productive employment* to the ever-increasing millions of people in those countries. Only a small proportion of the population in underdeveloped countries can be employed in the capital-intensive kind of industry. Most people continue in a very low-intensity, unmechanized kind of agriculture and have low standards of living, with all the health problems deriving from that low standard.

The main problems of health therefore are not the problems of pollution but the problems of poverty caused by the industrial growth of the West, and the fact that underdeveloped countries are still importing capital-intensive equipment instead of developing more autonomously within their own capabilities, in such a way as to give employment to everyone at the appropriate standard of productivity—employment in which the cost of providing a workplace is a cost appropriate to the country concerned.

El Batawi: Lord Ashby emphasized the physical aspects—environmental, pollution of air and water—and also the past history of biological pollution in industrial countries which resulted in communicable and infectious diseases. To a great extent I agree with Dr White. I would say that there *is* much pollution in developing countries, of the biological kind, leading to the transmission of disease through water, food and vectors. These same diseases occurred in industrial countries in the past. However, these diseases are known to be of single causation, with different precipitating and aggravating factors, but in general they are relatively easy to control. Diseases such as typhoid fever or cholera are simpler to control than the diseases of multiple aetiology associated with industrial growth. I would say, for example, that *psychosocial* 'pollution' is one of the important problems of modern societies and that diseases such as heart disease, hypertension, mental disorder, peptic ulcer, alcoholism and drug abuse have all been associated with such factors as industrial growth, the increasing speed of life, and the identification with machines and mechanical processes at the expense of human factors. The various types of psychosocial distress influence the health of societies to a great extent. They are influencing industrialized societies and are now starting to appear in developing countries.

Ashby: I agree, and I am sure that it is the destruction of institutions like the extended family, with its cohesion and assurance, that is among the losses that have followed the westernization of Africa. To what extent this is due to industry and not to education is a matter for discussion. I think the exporting of our educational systems with too little change has been a major cause, and I hope to extend this point later (see p. 214).

Mars: Lord Ashby made the point that in the hands of a corrupt inspectorate, the British system of pollution control could be disastrous. This is an important point. If we look at the British experience, the Industrial Revolution got going in Britain by 1800 and economic historians recognize that it was well established by 1850. But it was only then, in 1851, that we had the Northcote-Trevelyan Report which brought in a bureaucratic civil service without benefit of patronage and *laid the basis* for much of the factory and anti-pollution legislation we have now. This is not to deny, as Dr White said, that it is dangerous to take one country's experience and translate it to another—certainly not without taking into account the different time-scales and different cultural situations. But another and a related point to consider is whether there is some necessary sequence of social development before impartially administered pollution control *can* be effective. The first sequences of development in industrialization are often uncontrolled and there may well have to be a gap before the social prerequisites for impartial bureaucratized controls can begin to be introduced.

Ashby: Would you add that we may have exported some of our post-Northcote bureaucracy and to this extent we may have saved some trouble?

Mars: Yes, but many things can't be exported. I am thinking here of the problems that arise when innovation is guided by bureaucracies which are themselves modelled on an ideal—that relationships should be based on one strand—on the impartiality of contract. The reality is that many, though certainly not all, underdeveloped societies have a different basis for organizing their social relations. This basis often depends on the obligations of kinship or on other obligations that are personal rather than impersonal. And in many underdeveloped societies kinship is still an important factor. It is this that brings associated problems of what *we* would call corruption.

Phoon: It is true that we cannot extrapolate the experiences of one country and one situation directly to another country, but there are many similarities between what happened in Britain during the last century or so and what is happening in developing countries now. Moreover, there is no clear-cut demarcation between developed and developing countries. Not all developing countries are similar, and not all developed countries have equally developed sectors in their own territories. While it is true that in South-East Asia most countries are still largely agricultural and pollution is still mainly organic, within those countries, even the more backward ones, there are rapidly growing centres of urbanization and industrialization. The *pace* of such industrialization is very fast: changes which happened in a hundred years in the UK are happening in decades in some places. My own country, Singapore, is at first glance not a typical South-East Asian country, or a typical developing country; but in fact it is typical in many ways. Within the last ten years or so in Singapore we have seen a change from the disease pattern of so-called developing countries, where most of the deaths are due to infectious diseases, to a pattern like that of the West, and our largest killers now are cancer and cardiovascular disease. In other words, we have arrived at civilization! Similarly, in other parts of South-East Asia one finds in, say, Indonesia, areas which were largely agricultural and where now many of the hazards of urban living and pollution are arising. This symposium is therefore very timely. I don't accept that the lessons that the UK has learnt are not necessarily applicable, but we have to make adjustments in applying them.

It is often said that we are now living in one world, but sometimes it looks as though we are living in two worlds. Many people are very conscious of pollution in the UK and also anxious about what is happening in developing countries, but not all the companies based in developed countries which go to developing countries to set up factories have the same civic-mindedness. They may have high standards of safety and occupational health in their own countries, either by choice or by compulsion, but this is forgotten when they extend to developing countries. We have not only to educate people in developing countries but to educate industrialists who are exporting danger and pollution to those countries, sometimes deliberately trying to take advantage of less knowledgeable governments and people there. We hope public opinion will put pressure on such companies to adopt reasonable standards of safety and health in developing countries where they are now manufacturing more and more things, making use of the cheap labour.

Papanek: As Dr El Batawi has suggested, there are major problems in psychosocial pollution: the climbing suicide rate, increased violence and crime in big cities, drug abuse, alcoholism, stress, anxiety, cardiovascular diseases. To this can be added the withering away of the extended family, the breaking of kinship ties and the breakdown of social groups at work and play. Finally: alienation and existential *Angst*. But I feel that these are symptoms rather than causes. The main cause I believe to be the whole concept of a centralized or hierarchical order system. This sort of order system has been exported all over the world in the guise of 'efficiency' or as an accompaniment to 18th or 19th century colonialism. By now it has become a worldwide pattern, regardless of social, political or religious systems.

We now can see that centralization itself is inherently wrong but it is difficult—and education is largely responsible for this—to devise alternative order systems that are *not* highly centralized, autocratic or hierarchical. Such a system (be it the Central Committee of the USSR, the Roman Catholic Church, the joint chiefs of Staff of the United States, or a girls' Primary School in Botswana) is the main problem facing us.

Ramalingaswami: The question really is one of what pathway a country decides to take towards development. As Professor Phoon suggests, the tragedy is repeating itself daily—the historical tragedy of the developed in the developing countries. The Green Revolution that gave us so many hopes in India, for example, brought with it the problem that the farmer has become used to highly toxic cheap pesticides, and it is difficult to get him to change to more expensive but biodegradable pesticides. We are caught up now in a situation where the changeover will be costly. On the other hand, in developing countries everyone knows that the inputs that are required to reduce microbial pollution of the environment are enormous. If we have to provide protected water supplies to every town and village in India, it will cost a huge sum and will take long to accomplish, not to speak of waste and sewage disposal and the treatment of waste products. When one matches this against what looks like a short cut to a rapid pace of development through industrialization, one ends up in the national planning process by dividing a small cake into smaller segments. Nevertheless, I think a holistic approach *is* needed and a design for living in which we try to adjust the various competing demands on the resources, using, as Dr White said, the cheapest, most abundant and most valuable resource that developing countries have, namely *people*, and new strategies that involve the innovative skills of people in altering their environment for health promotion. This sounds idealistic but unless one begins to attack this on an eco-system basis—the complex of man in his environment—I am afraid we shall continue the historical tragedy that is in fact taking place all the time now.

Dickinson: I suspect that we have begun this symposium with the implicit assumption that the only way to get a higher quality of life is through industrialization of the western type, and that the problem therefore is of *how* we pass on to the naive the benefits of our sort of society. If this is our idea of aid, we can see why Development Decades go backwards rather than forwards! I suggest that if we look at this objectively, we shall see that other people have their own societies, their own organizations, and their own social structures; they decide their actions on the bases of their own social ambitions, on what they are prepared to sacrifice to achieve these ambitions, and on what they want in terms of health to suit *their* society, not ours. All we can do is to offer them the alternatives we know are possible, not forgetting the limitations that we have discovered by experience; but we must not presume that we can choose the things that are best for them. If we begin with humility about our ignorance, rather than certainty about our professional capacities, we may get further in providing genuine help.

References

1. MINISTRY OF AGRICULTURE, FISHERIES AND FOOD (1971) *Survey of Mercury in Food*, HMSO, London
2. REPORT OF THE STUDY OF CRITICAL ENVIRONMENTAL PROBLEMS (1970) *Man's Impact on the Global Environment*, MIT Press, Cambridge, Mass.
3. GOLDSMITH, E. *et al.* (1972) A blueprint for survival. *The Ecologist*, pp. 2-43, London
4. NEWMAN, J. H. (1872) *Discussions and Arguments on Various Subjects*, p. 293, Pickering, London
5. DERBY, LORD (Chairman) (1862) Report of the Select Committee appointed to study Noxious Vapours. Parliamentary Papers, Cmnd., HMSO, London
6. BEAVER, SIR H. (Chairman) (1954) Ministry of Housing and Local Government, Report of the Committee on Air Pollution. Cmnd. 9322, HMSO, London
7. ASHBY, SIR E. (Chairman) (1971-1973) Royal Commission on Environmental Pollution. First Report (Cmnd. 4585, 1971); Second Report (Cmnd. 4894, 1972); Third Report (Cmnd. 5084, 1972), HMSO, London
8. STANDING TECHNICAL COMMITTEE ON SYNTHETIC DETERGENTS (1958-1971) Progress Reports 1-12, Ministry of Housing and Local Government, HMSO, London
9. McLOUGHLIN, J. (1972) *The Law Relating to Pollution*, p. 112 (quoting Sturgess v. Bridgman (1897), 11, Ch. D. 856), Manchester University Press, Manchester
10. MALMESBURY, EARL OF (1884) *Memoirs of an Ex-Minister: an Autobiography*, vol. 2, p. 124, Longmans, Green, London

Legislative protection of health at work in the UK

J. C. WOOD

The regulation of conditions of work in the UK by legislation was one of the earliest examples of state intervention in private industry. It began, consequent upon the Industrial Revolution, early in the 19th century. The struggle to obtain and improve this legislative control is now an area of social history that has attracted considerable attention*. The early legislation was aimed at textile mills. It was much concerned with limiting hours of work and it dealt especially with children, young persons and women. Health aspects appeared right at the start but they were later to give second place to safety. The provisions for enforcement have always lagged behind the intentions and hopes of the legislature. Indeed it can still be argued today that the problem of effective enforcement remains a major issue. The earliest statute was enacted in 1802. The present current law is contained in several major statutes including the important Factories Act 1961.

The whole subject of health and safety at work has been the subject of a recent comprehensive review by the Robens Committee (1970–1972)[2]. The committee report does three things. It gives insight into the state of legislation in this area. It raises a large number of fundamental problems, of both major and minor consequences. It suggests a possible way forward. The first important steps have been taken by the passing of the Health and Safety at Work Act 1974. Plainly, the next few years are going to be a period of important reform and development. Most of these developments will be largely of domestic concern. They will nonetheless be reactions to underlying problems: problems which are of a wider and more fundamental nature. The first of these seems rather trivial, yet its importance cannot be ignored. The development of

---

* A good factual summary is to be found in ref. 1 (see p. 29). Social historians now attach considerable importance to this area of development.

the legislative code has been haphazard. Most often action has been taken as a result of social pressure upon a particular facet (for example, the early regulation of long hours), or has arisen from a tragedy or disaster*. This has led to a very uneven and illogical body of law. It has also led to control being spread among several government departments. It might be useful to examine this problem first.

CONTROL OF HEALTH AND SAFETY

The issues here are surprisingly complicated. Health and safety at work is very hard to confine between clear limits. The safety of the public is plainly an allied topic and immediately raises the issues of pollution and planning. These topics are a great deal wider, and immediately a problem of relationships is raised. The same applies to health. The very important task of the regulation of health is the concern of a major department of state. Occupational health lies naturally in the field of employment. Again, demarcation difficulties arise. Our experiences in the UK multiply this problem. The Home Office regards fire as its province: pollution, and so factory emissions, is a matter for the Department of the Environment: safety in mines and quarries concerns the Department of Trade and Industry. Although the paramountcy of the interests of the Department of Employment has been generally recognized the difficulties of the boundaries of the subject must not be minimized.

The Health and Safety at Work Act 1974 has attempted to meet this problem by the creation of an independent agency comprising a Health and Safety Commission and Executive (Section 9 of the Act). The Act sketches an outline of the new agency. The Robens Committee gave a more detailed indication of the likely organization[3]. There is evidence that there was considerable opposition among the various departments to this rationalization. In these proposals, the control of fire remains with the Home Office. Agriculture has managed, after some in-fighting, to remain outside the new framework, though a recent (September 1974) government consultative document proposes to reverse this. Two important principles emerge. The fragmentation of control is undesirable and contributes to incidents such as that at Dudgeons Wharf, where an explosion occurred when a tank farm was being dismantled[4]. Although there will always be demarcation problems a solid core of centralized direction is essential. Such steps should not, however, lessen concern for the need for

---

* Here there are very many important examples. Perhaps most remarkable was the death of eight in a mill fire at Keighley, which exposed the great weakness of the legislation concerning fire risks. This led to important provisions in the Factories Act, 1959.

effective communication with allied fields. This applies at all levels, and two were stressed by the Robens Committee: research, and regional and area executive action. This is an area in which the new Commission has much to do. It is of fundamental importance.

THE LEGAL FRAMEWORK

Perhaps the most unusual demand is for 'simple law in plain English'. This alas seems an unattainable objective. Nonetheless, the piecemeal growth of the topic has led to a very confused and inadequate framework of law. The Robens Committee proposed a simpler framework and stressed the need for flexibility so that the law could develop organically.

There are needs for three levels of law. Overall there needs to be a set of basic principles. These have developed both in the course of statutory control and also through the common law, especially that part of the law of negligence dealing with the liability of an employer. The 1974 Health and Safety at Work Act has begun this process. The old statutory emphasis upon types of premises—factory, workshop, office, shop and so on—has been replaced. There is a central emphasis upon the employment relationship. The duties are put in general terms upon the self-employed, the controller of premises, manufacturers and upon employees themselves (Sections 2–7 of the Act). The exact legal significance of the consolidation of the common law duties is far from clear. It should, however, mean that the inspectorate function can be exercised over a more general area.

The greatest mass of legal regulation is to be found in the corpus of statutory regulations*. Theoretically they form a detailed, responsive method of reacting to new dangers. In practice the methods of enactment and repeal are exceptionally slow, so the regulations fail to achieve the up-to-date protection that is ideally sought. This can be changed. It is perhaps more difficult to pitch regulations at a suitably strict level. Since they are of universal operation, except in instances of great risk, they tend to be pitched at a level all can easily achieve. Thus the best practice will quite often go beyond the regulatory demands.

It is here that the Code of Practice has its place. A Code can be flexible, recommending differing approaches and levels. It can spring more easily from examples of best practice. The Robens Committee laid great stress on the Code of Practice. It felt that such codes would enable the Inspectorate to use

---

* A handy collection of current regulations is to be found in the latest edition of Redgrave's *Factories Acts*[5].

constructively the Improvement Notice, a form of enforcement intended to achieve good safety standards before the situation leads to an accident. This approach attracted considerable criticism. It was felt by some to be weakening the impact of the law. Clearly, the right balance must be struck between general principle, regulation and code. The opposition to development through codes raises two fundamental problems. The relationship between enforcement and advice is called into question. It is also important to recognize the intricate relationship between safety regulation and accident compensation.

ENFORCEMENT OR ADVICE

One of the most difficult tasks is to achieve, in an area such as safety control, the right balance between advice and persuasion as against enforcement and sanctions. It is inevitable that groups that seek control of any particular area—planning, pollution, conservation, whatever it may be—tend to look for strong legislation and firm enforcement. Those not so enthusiastic tend to point out two weaknesses in this approach. There appears to be a limit to the level of achievement. Unless there is a strong desire for self-regulation, enforcement tends to be at the same time inadequate and onerous. Beyond a certain point only draconian enforcement will secure marginal improvement. Enforcement too tends to follow breach, which in the field of safety control is a paradox. The law seeks to prevent: enforcement tends to seize most readily upon breaches after accidents have happened. The attachment of many trade unionists and their theoretical supporters to this view[6] is somewhat ironic because in the field of industrial relations they argue strongly that legal regulation is not the best method to affect conduct and that strict enforcement by sanction is counter-productive.

This dilemma—or perhaps it should be described as the search for the correct balance between advice and enforcement—is the area where the enforcement agencies need to develop truly professional expertise. Their view seems basically to favour a consultative approach backed by necessary powers of sanction. Achieving a satisfactory balance is not at all easy.

COMPENSATION

In England, safety legislation has become very much the property of lawyers who specialize in compensation actions. This has arisen to a large extent because of the so-called action for breach of statutory duty. Under the doctrine it is possible for a person, injured through another's failure to act as a statute requires, to use this breach as a basis for an action for compensation. The action is to some extent parallel to that produced by the tort of negligence*.

It was argued in the Robens Report that the concentration upon the compensatory aspects of safety legislation has not always acted in the best interests of safety[7]. Certainly it means that a great deal of attention has been paid to the compensatory aspects of the subject. These, by their very nature, must be secondary to the basic aim of ensuring safety. There is considerable support for our present system, largely from those closely involved in it. Insurers stress, and almost certainly overstress, the effect of premium rates on safety provision. Trade unions assist their members to gain compensation and so see advantages. They tend to ignore the overall haphazard nature of the compensatory system†. Finally, the legal profession services the complicated rules and difficult legislation. The Robens Committee soon became aware of other ways of tackling this question. Of particular interest were the systems in British Columbia, Ontario and New Zealand. This area was outside the terms of reference of the Committee but it recommended further investigation.

Shortly after the Robens Report was published difficulties in the allied area of compensation for damage were raised in an acute and tragic way by the thalidomide affair. The result was the setting up of a Royal Commission under Lord Pearson to examine this area. Its Report, which is expected in 1975, will be of the greatest importance. The need to prevent compensation interfering with a logical structure of legislation, control, enforcement and, above all, investigation is of paramount importance.

HEALTH

A good example of the problems encountered in making provision for regulatory control is the topic of occupational health. The chapter on this subject in the Robens Report (chapter 12) is perhaps one of its weakest. Its weakness springs largely from the difficulties of the present situation. There are two approaches to the organization of occupational medicine. Those engaged chiefly in this field, whose views were put by the Society of Occupational Medicine, favour an extension of the work they are doing inside the structure of industry. There are indeed many examples of excellent work in industries with serious health hazards—the Atomic Energy Authority and firms processing asbestos—or with risk of serious injuries—the British Steel Corporation and

---

* Any good book on the law of tort deals fully with these matters—leading authors are Salmond, Winfield and Street. The latest edition of any of these books is a good source of a detailed summary of the principal features of the law.

† A leading academic critique has the title *The Forensic Lottery*[8]. For a more recent comprehensive review of the area, see ref. 9.

the National Coal Board. In addition, individual firms and doctors do important, and often pioneering, work on subjects such as noise or mental health. There is a very strong case for the encouragement of such developments.

There are, however, two snags. It has not been found easy to achieve parallel developments in smaller firms. Attempts to set up cooperative action, as at Slough, have not proved successful. Equally difficult is the feeling that in some areas the provision of medical facilities leads to waste of scarce qualified personnel. If active work is not being pressed forward, there tends to be little for the occupational health team to do. Routine doctoring is the prerogative of the family doctor. The monitoring of a worker's general health belongs to his home, rather than his work, environment. There will rarely be any connection between a firm's medical staff and the worker's family. Although it would be possible to change this, and Eastern European countries offer possible models, the provision of family medicine by a general practitioner is thought by many doctors to be the keystone of our system of medical provision.

It follows that there is a countervailing body of medical opinion which, while recognizing the importance of factory-based medicine, sees the most important way forward as the introduction of an occupational medicine specialty into the growing number of 'group practices'. The emphasis on occupational medicine problems in family medicine is obviously an important gain. There remain, however, real difficulties. The general practitioner with a large case-load—and each patient who works has a potentially different work environment—is presented with a really difficult task of measuring symptoms against a background which is only appreciated by perhaps inaccurate description.

There is also suspicion of administrative problems too. The old 'factory doctor' who has been a feature of legislation for a long time was largely concerned with the strength and fitness of young persons for work. The legislative move to an employment medical advisory service was a recognition of work begun by the medical inspectorate*. This development has been confirmed in the 1974 Act. There seems, however, to be a lack of parallel and integrated development in the National Health Service, which is of course the responsibility of the Department of Health and Social Security.

It is not necessary to go into greater detail to establish the main problems. There is an important and increasing role for the expert in occupational medicine. New techniques, the use of fresh chemicals, the greater awareness of problems such as noise and mental health, all point to the need for real effort in this field. It is hard, however, to be sure in which direction this effort should

---

* See the Employment Medical Advisory Service Act 1972.

be made. The history and current organization of general medicine have an inevitable effect on the potential for the development of occupational medicine. It is essential to accept that progress can only be made if the constraints of the surrounding, well-established social background are recognized.

GENERAL COMMENTS

It will be obvious from what has been said that the area of health and safety at work is one in which problems abound. Many of them raise points of fundamental importance, which are extremely difficult to resolve. An example is the part to be played by the work-force in safety. It is beyond doubt that the psychological perspective is of paramount importance. A man's safety depends upon engineering, planning of work and so on. But it also depends to a very large extent on his own desire for safety, his attention to safety, and his constant mental awareness. It follows that the attitude of trade unions and of each individual worker is crucial. Trade unions certainly say that they are extremely devoted to the topic, but their record does not always show firm and consistent enthusiasm. It is here, perhaps, that most can be done: the individual workmen's reaction to safety training, to the proffered safety devices, and to managerial supervision of safety aspects. It follows that anything which increases the involvement of workers in this area is to be welcomed. The first bill, introduced by the Conservative Government*, was substantially altered by the succeeding Labour Government on this point and the 1974 Act provides for both worker safety representatives and safety committees in specified areas.

Of equal difficulty is the practical application of the undoubted truth that anyone with line management responsibilities must have a responsibility for safety. How to ensure continuous awareness of this responsibility is not easy. In the USA it is quite usual for the position to be reinforced by loss of bonus. It is doubtful whether such an approach could easily be transplanted. Yet it is essential that some method be used which is appropriate to and effective in the particular society. There are two real difficulties. One is that the pressure for production, particularly where delivery dates are pressing, can so easily outweigh the need for vigilance on safety. Similar dangers arise where emergencies occur. Attention is turned towards the particular problem and unless there has been careful forethought on procedures and training to ensure safe reflexes, accidents happen. A difficulty of similar importance is the exact use to be made of specialist safety staff. Where the size of the firm warrants it, specialized staff are essential. But they cannot be used to absolve others of

---

* The bill lapsed at the February 1974 dissolution of Parliament.

responsibility. The manager should be able to use these specialized resources but his overall, basic responsibility must not be obscured. Equally, the natural and enthusiastic pressure for an improved professionalism for safety specialists (epitomized by the good work done by the Institution of Industrial Safety Officers) should not close the area to those in general management who might at some stage of their careers be willing to spend a period in the field of safety.

These are but examples of the type of challenging issue that presents itself to those trying to improve the structure and institutions aiming at safety. There are very many other such problems.

Overall, unhappily, the real enemies are apathy, thoughtlessness and boredom. The subject of safety has little sensational interest—in this it differs so markedly from, for example, industrial relations. It is not a subject that can be pursued for a while and then left on one side for a while. Inconsistent attention is dangerous. The subject is one which requires steady and consistent effort. The Health and Safety at Work Act 1974 should give a boost to English attention to the area. Efficiency demands a five-year programme of reform. The new Authority means that there is a very important task of creating a new, effective piece of administrative machinery. All this is challenging, if not exciting. Yet health and safety ultimately depend on the concern and awareness of the individual worker or manager. If this can be aroused and maintained, improvement will be inevitable.

Discussion

El Batawi: Professor Wood touched on many points that we are keenly interested in at WHO, particularly the question of fragmentation of effort in the health field. Man is contained within one body and health is a totality, yet, because of historical factors and the evolution of public health disciplines independently from the labour movement and labour protective legislation, industrial medicine tended to be regarded as a separate field that may or may not be integrated with general health services, depending on political and other factors. In many countries health services to workers are often fragmented and implemented by several authorities, with low effectiveness and limited achievements.

There is also a problem of the inadequacy of legislation—its incomplete coverage of the working population, particularly in small-scale industries. For these and other reasons the approach that WHO follows and is trying to communicate to developing countries is to consider occupational health as an integral part of the countries' health services. General practitioners should be educated in occupational health so they can bring more effective preventive services to workers. At the same time occupational health practitioners should care for the general health problems of the workers and not limit their work to the narrower scope of occupational disease problems. Our last Expert Committee Report emphasizes that occupational health is an integral part of public health. It also refers to the special problems of small-scale industries and emphasizes the close relations between occupational health and public health[10]. We don't want to see a demarcation line between the public health centre and the occupational centre; we don't want to say that the worker's health is the responsibility of the employer alone. It is the responsibility of society, because employees are affected by general diseases, in addition to disabilities related to their work.

Bridger: Everyone would agree that we should consider the whole aspect of affairs, just as we should consider the whole man and not merely symptoms and isolated behaviour. But we need to understand why this tendency to fragmentation exists and the processes that comprise it. If not, the size of the problem could lead us to the cynical approach of Machiavelli: those attempting to innovate change will have for enemies those who benefited under the old system and will only have lukewarm support from those who think the new ideas might work! We have to face the problem of how far it is possible to develop multidisciplinary or multifunctional and integrative processes among people, or among groups, or among government departments. This will not be found to be so popular in practice as it is in theory. Integrative processes cannot be achieved simply on a *rational* basis. Many such attempts are doomed when it is decided to work in those modes that do not include emotive aspects. *Intellectually* we can appreciate and grasp far more in a situation than we are capable of handling in attempting to adapt to the change as a real-life experience. These adaptive processes entail involving ourselves in the problems of relationships—role and institutional relationships as well as inter- and intrapersonal ones. Our inability to give sufficient attention to facing and understanding these human processes is probably the greatest stumbling block to the integration of ideas, people, technologies, structures and other resources.

It is when we begin to recognize some of the factors affecting *ourselves* that we can begin to identify and work through problems inherent in our own situation. The processes involved, and not just the accumulation of data, must be a *primary* consideration and not something to bear in mind.

Wood: Dr El Batawi rather frightens me by synthesizing everything: everything that could possibly be done is integrated within his encapsulated scheme. In my paper I was trying to say that this approach just won't work. We have tried to get British industries to cooperate on health and safety but they are far too independent and too established in their ways to do this. Dr El Batawi's integrated approach to health and safety might work in a green-field site, but not in an established industry. One has indeed to recognize Machiavelli's point and to approach the situation by removing the barriers preventing people from developing in the way one wants them to go. That is what we have done with the new Health and Safety Authority in the UK. As long as alkali control is in one department and factory control in another, they will grow apart and build walls between themselves. Put them together and they may hate it, but their successors will not remember that they were in separate departments, so you will have *removed* the pressures. I approve of academic blueprints but one has to recognize that that is what they are, and having looked at them, it is necessary to ask what walls can be knocked down so that people *themselves* move into the new desired patterns.

It is the same with industrial compensation. One would have to persuade the insurance companies, the lawyers and the trade unions that it is in their *own* interests to develop in the way we think they should go. This is what Royal Commissions are about. They are not about quick legislation; they are about knocking down barriers, moving things, so that people want to go in the way it is thought they should go.

Jones: I see a contradiction between your argument in favour of bringing down barriers and the other possible anxiety about giving people *too much* information, which makes issues emotive, and this is uncomfortable for lawyers! I can't see how one will get the degree of cooperation, let alone the necessary motivation, unless people are given the necessary information.

Wood: The giving of information raises enormous problems. As soon as you start making statements that, say, the patient's temperature today is 99 °F, people start doing things, and they are then acting because of your information; if it turns out badly, they are off to their lawyers. It therefore raises problems.

Jones: I appreciate the dilemma. If for the last 20 years, for example, we had had the cooperation and employee involvement proposed under the new Health and Safety at Work Act, would we, in a vinyl chloride plant, with our present knowledge about its carcinogenicity, still be able to retain the confidence and the principle of voluntary enforcement by the employees? Couldn't they quite cynically say that you involved us all that time ago but didn't tell us, forgetting that 20 years ago we didn't know of the existence of this new risk?

Wood: That is right; but if we take the problem further back to the person who has to evaluate the rumour or the suspicion or the information, at what stage does he have to pass this on to people? He has then an enormous personal dilemma: should he tell people at the first possible moment, which could be scare-mongering, or should he tell them at the last permissible moment, which may be careless?

Bridger: There is always the crucial problem of learning how to balance and regulate physical and social systems: we know, for example, that fire or water have their values and also their dangers. In fact, we are beginning to recognize that today many systems are really out of control. Our chances of dealing effectively with such situations depend on facing these issues and not pretending otherwise. Then, any steps in the direction of resolving conditions entails balancing and optimizing the various conflicting objectives and the internal forces, which will be far from congruent. First and foremost we have to create the kind of climate which will permit such balancing and optimizing to take place. I can sympathize here with Dr Papanek, who mentioned hierarchies (p. 13). What kinds of structures are appropriate to certain objectives? How do you *lead* people in situations where interdependence is the appropriate approach? How do you deal with those many situations in community and organizational life where one cannot have creativity without destructiveness? This is not just a psychological point; it is a practical operational matter. We need to recognize that in addition to attaining overt objectives we have, as a corresponding, complementary task, to spend time and effort on the *ways* in which we are working and in the forces operating them.

Papanek: On the matter of giving information, I don't think we can assume any longer that confidentiality and classified information can still exist. All information is becoming de-classified; there is almost no choice in the situation now, and the concept of confidentiality of any kind of consumer information or labour information or health information is vanishing. I personally welcome that.

Gilson: I would like to continue the point of how we can learn from our mistakes, in relation to the asbestos problem. The problem of asbestosis was discovered in the UK and in the US in the 1930's; actions were taken to improve the situation within the knowledge of the then technology. Evidence of cancer associated with asbestos working was already appearing in the early 1940's, but action was not taken, because of the fragmentation of information. Had there been continuous research into the data accumulating after 1930 (as was proposed by the Chief Medical Inspector of Factories), perhaps things would have been different today. Technology changed; regulations did not keep up. There is one way in which the developed countries can contribute on a worldwide basis which is not possible in developing countries—namely, by seeing that their national records are used to monitor new and assess old occupational hazards.

El Batawi: Professor Wood referred to my earlier comment as an academic blueprint that may not work—at least not in the UK! This may be true, because of the walls that have been built between different health systems that are dealing in one way or another with workers' health. In the developing countries we are still at a point where we can do something and establish sound integrated comprehensive health services for workers. When I said that occupational physicians should be trained in public health, so that they may have a comprehensive approach to health, this *is* being practised by Professor Phoon, for example, who is giving a course in occupational medicine, particularly emphasizing public health aspects. In developing countries we are trying to avoid segregated, ineffective programmes; we have inherited a good deal of it from colonial times, and we are trying to get a holistic approach established and to deal with human health as a totality.

Challis: Large industrial firms tend to be used as examples of both good and bad practice, but even very large firms, strangely enough, are made up of people, and in the end, no matter how big an organization may be, its attitude to safety, welfare, pollution and production comes down to a question of people's emotions and their morality. That is an old-fashioned word but it does mean something. For example, take the question of production *versus* safety. Trade unions, when they want a wage increase, often argue that the management will throw safety to the winds when the firm wants high levels of production in order to make a profit. They imply that their members regard safe working as an absolute requirement of the job—and a reasonable employer would agree with that sentiment. In the next negotiation, there may well be a claim for 50 pence an hour 'danger money', which is an interesting reflection on both morality and the emotional approach to problems. On the other hand, the management of a firm often counter accusations of unsafe working by saying: 'look at the laws we have to work under and the safety codes that we have'. Yet the *reality* is that people under pressure cut corners, and the real safety of an operation depends more upon the attitudes of people than upon codes. We free ourselves in industry of some of the worst mistakes if we can explain to people that of course they are human, and they have to look at their mistakes and their corner-cutting, learn the lessons of over-enthusiasm and *relax* a little. This may be a useful thing for the less-developed industrial nations to bear in mind, because by taking that attitude you try to avoid massive confrontation between regulatory authorities and those being regulated, and to encourage groups of people—management and men—to do something which goes along a moral path.

Finally, at the end of it all, you have to decide what is the minimum you are prepared to let people get away with, in health, safety, or anything else, and you then introduce a draconian regulation at that point. If you put such regulations into force at a fairly tolerable level the measure will be accepted, because the average man in industry will accept its reasonableness. However, if you put in, as the Americans have done in some fields, a very high standard of regulation and apply draconian measures, there will be great resentment, and resentment means dodging the issue.

In dealing with all matters of legal enforcement of standards, one must constantly keep in mind the desired objective. This is a high standard of safety or health for the people who are being subject to the law. The *way* in which this objective is achieved is less important than the fact that it is being achieved. A colleague of mine uses the phrase 'tolerance of ambiguity', and it is a useful one to bear in mind when we consider how legislation can be made to work. A lower legal standard that is accepted is more valuable than a 'tough' regulation which is evaded. Engage people's emotions and the battle is half won. This is something that industry is often bad at, because we have been technically trained, a bit like lawyers, to lay out problems clearly and logically. We then expect that because someone understands the logic he will follow the prescription. This just doesn't happen often for other, *emotional* reasons. Laws and regulations are excellent, but only as a means to an end: safer working or better health.

A final point is that we need to realize that the problems we are discussing are rooted back in human beings and that the technical manager with a degree is an ordinary human being when he goes home to his wife, the same as the production worker on the shop floor; both have the same problems of emotion. The main point to concentrate on, in looking at the WHO blueprint, is how one makes it work. The British method has its defects but it works, at least in the UK. It may not be the only way of using regulations to improve health and safety, but it has as its basis the recognition that people are not all angels, and that if we encourage people when they are staggering out from a low level of health and safety practices, they will progress further.

Wood: The American system of building into individual managers (line managers) a system by which they lose their bonuses if they have accidents was examined by the Robens Committee and we decided that it wouldn't transplant into the British trade union situation.

References

1. HUTCHINS, B. L. & HARRISON, A. (1966) *A History of Factory Legislation*, Cass, London
2. ROBENS, LORD (Chairman) (1972) *Safety and Health at Work*. Report of the Committee 1970-72, Cmnd. 5034, HMSO, London
3. See ref. 2, especially chapter 4 (pp. 31-39) and the chart on p. 71
4. *Report of Public Inquiry into a Fire at Dudgeons Wharf on 17th July 1969*, Cmnd. 4470, HMSO, London (1970)

5. REDGRAVE, A. (1972) *Factories Acts*, 22nd edn, Butterworth, London
6. SIMPSON, R. C. (1973) Safety and Health at Work: Report of the Robens Committee 1970-72. *36 Modern Law Review*, 192
7. See ref. 2, Appendix 7
8. ISON, T. G. (1967) *The Forensic Lottery*, Staples Press, London
9. ATIYAH, P. S. (1970) *Accidents, Compensation and the Law*, Weidenfeld & Nicolson, London
10. WORLD HEALTH ORGANIZATION (1973) Environmental and health monitoring in occupational health. *Technical Report Series* no. 535

Lessen the industrial growing pains of developing countries by more effective aid

N. Y. KIROV

INTRODUCTION: HOW THE OTHER HALF LIVES

Industrial growth has helped to create an immense inequality between the nations of the world, and the gap continues to widen. The poorer half of the world's population earns only 7% of the world income and averages an annual income of less than £25 per head.

To belong to an underdeveloped or developing country means to be poor; it means that one needs to be tougher to survive than in developed countries—infant mortality up to one year of age is greater. It means spending a large part of one's life being rather hungry; it means inadequate diet and malnutrition, and this leads to poor health under conditions of inadequate medical care; it also means sub-standard education, limited job opportunities, low productivity and low income, employment insecurity and, finally, a shorter life (for example, the life expectancy for a five-year-old girl in the UK or USA is 71 years, whereas in India it is 47, in Burma 50 years).

What image do developing countries see of their future? To them, rising material standards mean a better and happier life, the availability of work, better working conditions, less hunger, better housing, improved health, the opportunity for wider education, more security in life. It is true that environmental pollution and wastes generally accompany technological developments, but these problems are insignificant compared with the benefits technology can confer.

'Between 40 and 70% of the developing world's 2000 million people live below the poverty line, and at least 40% of them live in absolute poverty', the UN Commission on Human Rights was told recently. 'Despite a decade of unprecedented increase in gross national product, the poorest segments of the population of the less developed lands survive on incomes of about 20 cents a

31

day'. It is estimated that two-thirds of the population of underdeveloped countries is suffering from malnutrition. Hence, the immediate concern of these countries is not with 'Health and Industrial Growth', but rather with the necessity to provide employment for their growing populations, and to develop what industries they can, and as soon as they can, in order to prevent widespread disease, hunger and unemployment.

Industrialize they must, but by applying what kind of technology? And, in applying it, how best can they learn from the mistakes and experience of the developed countries? It is in providing answers to such questions, perhaps, that the developed countries can really help.

INDUSTRIAL DEVELOPMENT AND THE ENVIRONMENT

Environmental degradation is essentially a problem of people: we associate it with the activities of man; it is a problem of large cities and of modern affluent society, of a wasteful consumer economy and the indiscriminate use of dwindling natural resources.

In attempting to diagnose the problem in the developed (and the developing) countries, one may ask: where does the blame (*culpa*) lie, then, for the dangers (*pericula*, perils) arising from the exponential growth of pollution and environmental degradation? The answer is contained in the following equation:

$$(PED)^e = E^2 = PERILS\ CULPI^n$$

The first part of this equation provides a reminder that the *E*ffluent *E*xplosion (E^2) and the benefits of technological development are generally accompanied by an almost exponential growth of *P*ollution and *E*nvironmental *D*egradation $(PED)^e$. The effect on the environment is compounded by the following major factors:

*P*opulation	*C*ars ($\equiv$ modern transport)
*E*xplosion	*U*rbanization (city growth)
*R*ising	*L*ack of
*I*ndustrialization, and	*P*lanning
*L*iving	*I*gnorance (and negligence to the *n*th
*S*tandards	degree)

The Population Explosion is 'everybody's baby' and most scientists would generally agree that overpopulation gives today the greatest cause of concern, particularly in the underdeveloped and developing countries.

Rising industrialization and living standards

Today's industrialized nations have become geared to a philosophy of growth and rising material standards of living. Such societies are growing rapidly and making increasingly greater demands on finite world resources.

This unprecedented growth in the demand on natural resources obviously cannot be sustained for long. It certainly cannot be extended to other regions of the globe without the world outgrowing its non-renewable resources. Pressures from impending shortages are already in evidence. Many of these resources come from undeveloped and developing countries which, too, aspire to reach the level of industrialization of the 'advanced' countries and may in future withhold these resources in order to meet their own growing demands and safeguard their future needs.

There is already evidence of growing unrest in some areas, with countries becoming aware of their bargaining strength (for example, the oil-exporting countries). This may well be a cause for future world conflicts.

The amount of energy used in different countries is in some way related to the achieving of a given level of gross national product (GNP), and while rising material standards do not necessarily enhance the quality of life, rates of fuel consumption are often used as an index of living standards.

Such data as are available serve to emphasize the wide differences between developed and developing countries. At present a small fraction of the world's population consumes the greater part of its energy. In fact, North America, Western Europe, the Communist block (excluding China), South Africa, Japan and Australia consume over 90% of the world's energy, while the remaining 50% of the world population shares less than $7\frac{1}{2}$%.

The motor car

Symbolizing the development of modern transportation, the car is not only responsible for a large consumption of premium fuels but is also the major contributor to air pollution in urban areas. Car emissions are blamed for up to 60% of the total air pollutants in some of the large cities of the world.

Urbanization: the rapid growth of cities

Industrialization, with its promises of better economic opportunities, has lured people away from rural living. In 1920 only 14% of the world population was urban; this increased to 25% by 1960, and it is estimated that by the year 2000, 44% of the population will live in urban areas.

Figures for the US are even more dramatic: whereas in 1790, 95% of the population was rural, by 2000 about 85% is expected to be urban. And, in spite of its vast expanse of land and its comparatively small population, Australia has emerged as the most urban nation in the world, with 88.5% of its population living in cities at the end of 1970.

Thus, in the relatively short time since the Industrial Revolution of the mid-19th century, the large city has become the most characteristic form of modern social life. It is not surprising, therefore, that many mistakes have been made and that man is still learning to build large city communities, and to live happily in them.

To give but one example—Saigon. This is an attractive city of some three million people, once named the 'Paris of the Orient'. Traffic on its narrow, tree-lined streets has already reached saturation point, yet its western planners envisage that by the year 2000 it will have a population variously estimated at between 9.2 and 12.6 million people!

Lack of planning

Fragmentation of responsibilities between numerous authorities and preoccupation with the many problems arising from rapid population and industrial and urban growths have allowed little time for comprehensive and forward planning. This has resulted in piecemeal uncoordinated developments which do not provide an overall solution; frequently they result in new problems.

There is now an urgent need to plan on a long-term and comprehensive basis.

Ignorance and negligence to the nth degree

The effort made so far to prevent the growth and worsening of these problems has been completely inadequate. There is at present a lack of information about the full long-term effects and consequences of our actions. This is not an emotional issue and such policies as are needed must be based on facts. Yet, even the best available data for planning are just not good enough. We need more trained people, more equipment, more data collection and surveys, more applied research and development, and more personal involvement with such problems.

A WORLD DIVIDED: THE DRIFT APART

The inequality gaps between the developed and the developing countries, and within the developing countries themselves, are widening on many fronts. If this symposium can help to narrow some of these gaps through encouraging better understanding and more effective aid, it will have been worth while.

The population gap

Population concentrations and growth are greatest in those areas of the world which are least capable of providing for them. In India, for example, in spite of a well-established, government-sponsored family planning organization and a mass sterilization programme, the population is now increasing by one million every twenty-five days.

According to current UN statistics, the world's population increased by 76 million in the year to mid-1972, when it stood at 3782 million. More than half of the total (57% or 2154 million people) live in Asia. In other words, one out of every two people is an Asian, and the population growth in Asian countries is greater than that of the rest of the world—they accounted for 50 million of the 76 million increase in world population in 1972.

It is widely accepted that, short of an unforeseen world calamity, the world population cannot level off below 7000 million people. However, if effective control measures were taken now, it might be made to level off at about that figure, at which it could possibly be sustained in the future.

The gap between growth of GNP and consumption of resources

The world's natural mineral resources are irreplaceable, and must be used with restraint for the benefit of all nations if future conflicts and world tensions are to be avoided. From now on developed countries will have to make major decisions in terms of the overall quality of life, rather than in terms of standards of living and growth of GNP, as they do at present.

Today, the growth of incomes and productivity in the developing countries is partly offset by the high rate of population growth and by inequalities in incomes. For example, in a recent report of the World Bank, 39 developing countries were reviewed and it was shown that the top 5% of the population received 30 times more income than the lowest 40%.

In these countries energy consumption per head will have to be increased by 10 to 15 times to power the machines needed to produce enough food for their peoples. At present their energy consumption is well below the world average.

The educational and technological gap

This problem is being compounded by the lack of technical manpower and equipment and by the inability of governments to cope with the large and growing proportion of young people, who are making an increasing demand on inadequate and already overloaded education systems.

This is an area in which the developed countries have already provided some assistance. There is, however, scope for much more effective aid through teachers having technical skills and a sense of dedication—that is, by 'technological missionaries' who can successfully apply their skills to practical problems.

If we accept the fact that we must have industrialization in order to survive, the question then arises: what kind of industrial development is best for the Third World? Some would argue that it would be wrong to give the Third World an industrial production system similar to that of the developed countries, since this has largely been responsible for the mess they now find themselves in.

The concept of 'intermediate technology' (an unfortunate choice of words), originally put forward as a solution for the economic problems of India, appears promising and worth considering. This aims to develop and introduce techniques appropriate to the skills, resources and needs of a particular community. In the energy field, for example, intermediate technology would include the development of wind power, small-scale solar energy, small-scale water power, and animal- and vegetable-generated methane. This is because high productivity in agriculture is strongly energy-intensive.

The communication and credibility gap

Developing countries view all advice offered from developed countries with mistrust, and they will continue to do so as long as the developed countries worship industrial growth and plan for further expansion by staking claims on diminishing world resources.

Some underdeveloped countries have vast health problems beside which the adverse effects on health of industrial pollutants are insignificant. For example, the Asian country with which the developed countries have had the closest contact—South Vietnam—ranks first in the world with more than three million cases of venereal diseases (according to a survey published early in 1974). Thailand occupies second place on the list, with 600 000 cases.

Easier travel and closer contacts have not removed the communication gap or produced a better understanding of the problems of other nations. More tolerance, idealism and 'give and take' are needed to overcome prejudices and avoid future conflicts between nations.

INDUSTRIAL DEVELOPMENT: IS THERE A THREAT TO HEALTH?

In many parts of the world, industrial development has resulted in significant levels of contamination and environmental pollution. This problem, if left unchecked, will threaten our very existence. The World Health Organization warns: 'No environmental health problem has greater significance than the disposal of man's liquid and solid wastes'. In this regard, our concern should be with the total environment: noise and odour, water supply and sewage disposal, traffic flow and urban development, public health and comfort—all these are closely interrelated with land, air and water pollution problems and to a large extent are indivisible. In a finite world, they have become matters of international scope and concern, for pollution recognizes no national boundaries.

Serious air pollution, hazardous to health, is already occurring in most of the developing countries. Often it is due to the concentration of large industrial complexes in low-lying flat areas and along river valleys, with natural ventilation corridors through densely populated urban areas; the low-level discharge of smoke; the burning of cheap fuels with a high content of sulphur; poor plant maintenance; a lack of effective control of pollution at source; and the inadequate provision of pollution-control equipment. For example, Bien Hoa Industrial Park near Saigon contains 128 plants in various stages of construction or production, and is likely to become a major source of air and water pollution.

It is important to stress that it is the local concentrations of dangerous pollutants that are of significance for health, not the frequently quoted annual averages over a large area. The following examples of serious pollution are based on my own experience while working with the WHO.

Kaohsiung (Central Taiwan) is a centre of intensive industrial development. In 1971 the concentration of 14.3 parts per hundred million of sulphur dioxide in the air was already quite high (the WHO long-term recommended annual average is 2 p.p.h.m.). Yet, it is expected that by 1975 additional power plant capacity, burning 4% sulphur fuel oil, will be commissioned. In addition it was planned to construct a fertilizer and chemical works, copper roasting and refining, and heavy iron and steel industries. One can foresee here the creation of a serious problem of pollution.

At *Chin-Qua-Shih (Taipei County, Taiwan)* the Taiwan Metal Mining Corporation roasts sulphide ore to produce copper, silver and gold, and in so doing discharges daily up to 20 tons of sulphur dioxide at low level. In nearby dormitories live 3000 employees and their families. There is much sickness among the employees, yet the company plans a three-fold expansion of these activities.

At *Linkou* (*Taiwan*), the Taiwan power station discharges about 300 tons per day of sulphur dioxide from 12 chimneys of about 15 metres in height, serving fuel-oil-burning diesel units. Vegetation and trees in the surrounding area are badly affected, many chickens have died, and people in the nearby dormitories and village frequently complain of discomfort and inability to sleep at night. Spot readings of sulphur dioxide taken in December 1971 at the diesel office were 350 p.p.h.m. at 9.00 a.m. and 324 p.p.h.m. at 10.00 a.m.; and in the nearby dormitory areas the reading was 13 p.p.h.m. of sulphur dioxide. Such concentrations are hazardous to health.

In the *Nan Kang District* (*Taipei City, Taiwan*) the monthly average of fine suspended solids for October 1971 was 750.4 micrograms per cubic metre and this was accompanied by significantly high levels of sulphur dioxide. (For comparison, during the five-day smog disaster in London in 1952 to which 4000 excess deaths were attributed, a particulates concentration of 750 micrograms per cubic metre and a sulphur dioxide concentration of 25 p.p.h.m. were reported.)

In *Korea*, road transport and the Ondol domestic heating system are responsible for dangerous, and often fatal, concentrations of carbon monoxide. In Seoul and Taegu average concentrations for the period July–November 1970 were 33 p.p.m., with individual concentrations for two-hourly periods of up to 71.5 p.p.m. These are very high values, if we consider that the recommended long-term goal of WHO, not to be exceeded more than once a year, is 9 p.p.m. for an eight-hour period.

The unsolved problem of the domestic Ondol heating system is, however, much more serious. The floors of many Korean houses are provided with in-built horizontal flues, connected at one end to a fire-place and at the other end to a short chimney. Anthracite briquette fuel is commonly burnt, the hot flue gases providing household heating in winter. Unfortunately, substantial quantities of carbon monoxide are produced, which sometimes leak out into the living areas, with tragic consequences.

In 1969, there were 24 000 reported cases of carbon monoxide poisoning, with 1200 deaths. In 1971, 16 128 people were slightly affected, 5426 badly affected and 832 killed by carbon monoxide from these domestic fires. This is a far greater loss of life than that claimed by some of the more feared diseases.

The lack of an easily measurable and sensitive biological indicator is a serious limitation in ascertaining the effects on health of low-levels of pollution. However, evidence is accumulating that air pollution causes, or aggravates, diseases such as chronic bronchitis, pulmonary emphysema and lung cancer. There is evidence too that such diseases are on the increase in the developing countries.

In *Taiwan* cancer now ranks as the second most frequent cause of death, having increased by 40% over the period 1964–1970. The five areas most frequently subject to cancer are, in decreasing order of importance: stomach; lung; trachea and bronchi; intestine; mouth and throat; and oesophagus.

In *Saigon*, air pollution causes discomfort, soils clothes and affects eyes, throat and respiratory organs. In recent years many of the trees lining the narrow streets of the city have died and have had to be removed. Numerically, cases of respiratory diseases in the city hospitals are second only to those resulting from war casualties. Overcrowding of the narrow streets, congested traffic, tall buildings and lack of adequate parks and open areas, together with unfavourable meteorological conditions which restrict the normal dispersing and cleansing action of the atmosphere, all combine to produce serious pollution. Heavy emissions from the city's 200 000 old and badly maintained motor vehicles and over 400 000 motorized bicycles and motor-cycles were much in evidence, suggesting that ground levels of carbon monoxide in the major city thoroughfares were many times greater than those considered safe for health. Unfortunately, so far measurements of these pollution levels have not been made.

All these problems are likely to become worse before effective control measures are implemented.

SHOULD THE DEVELOPED COUNTRIES PROVIDE AID?

If it is agreed

(*i*)   That underdeveloped countries must develop technologically;

(*ii*) That, in so doing, health and industrial growth should not be in conflict; rather, they should develop in collaboration;

(*iii*) That this could be achieved by good planning and engineering, since the technology already exists; and

(*iv*) That they need assistance from the developed countries,

the question arises: *why* should the developed countries help?

Has the international community an obligation towards the developing countries? Has it a real concern about the effects on health arising from un-controlled industrial activities? Or is its concern only that in so developing, these countries may add to the demand on already dwindling resources of raw materials, many of which are within their own boundaries?

Ideally, one would like to think that such assistance by the developed countries would be motivated by purely unselfish, moral and humanitarian reasons, but human nature being what it is, reliance on such motivation would make effective aid an extremely slow process. However, there are other incentives, based on man's self-interest and his instinct for self-preservation.

It could be argued that aid so motivated is not a sacrifice but an investment in building a better world and improving the quality of life for all, including that of the already developed countries. World tensions, gross inequalities and environmental pollution are a threat to us all, and to help others develop is a cheaper and more effective way of helping ourselves in the long run. Developing countries will thus cease to be a liability and become an asset. Greater efficiency and improved productivity and product quality should pave the way to better labour relations, more purchasing power and improved international trade. Better utilization and more equitable distribution of diminishing world re-sources should lessen international tensions, and reduce the waste of resources on the manufacture of weapons of destruction. Environmental protection and effective control of pollution should improve health and make countries more attractive for tourism.

And if all this sounds too difficult and utopian to strive for, the alternatives are too dismal to contemplate.

TOWARDS MORE EFFECTIVE AID

'Bring fish to a poor man and you give him food for a day; give him a fishing rod and teach that poor man to fish, and he will not want for food'.

In many respects the technological aid provided to developing countries so far has been both insufficient and inefficient. Much effort has been wasted in supporting unpopular, weak and corrupt administrations—in supplying them with weapons of war and encouraging divisiveness, or in developing industries to suit the country providing the assistance, with little regard to the needs of the recipient country. A high proportion of the funds is currently being spent on advisers and planners working in splendid isolation, trying unrealistically to pattern the industrial production system of the Third World on the tech-nology of the developed countries. Emphasis is being placed on curing the disease and ill-effects of uncontrolled development rather than on safeguarding man's health and social well-being by good planning and engineering.

The modern concept of environmental health requires not merely the abatement of problems and nuisances, but also their prevention. In this respect much can be done to assist developing countries by the improved education and training of technical personnel; by the study of meteorological conditions and by taking these into account in the location of cities, green areas, power plants and factories; by the correct design and operation of industrial plant; by assisting in establishing those technologies which are most needed for the balanced development of the country; by the assessment and control of pollutants from various chemical processes; by subsidizing and encouraging the local manufacture of pollution-control equipment and of equipment needed to intensify primary production and local industries; and by helping to establish the necessary legislation, resources and organization for technical and engineering control and assistance.

All this requires a systematic approach, in order to identify and solve old and new problems. Modern technology is adequate for their solution but frequently it cannot be applied, because of a lack of the necessary resources or organization. Aid, properly conceived, is a supplement to the efforts of the developing countries towards economic development and eventual self-sustained growth. One way of making aid more effective is to provide it on a regional basis. Cooperation and the exchange of information and experience within a region are of value in solving some of these problems, particularly with poor countries which cannot afford individual programmes. International agencies can play an important role in promoting such regional cooperation. To give but one instance: in May 1973 the Regional Office for the Western Pacific of the WHO held its First Regional Seminar on Environmental Pollution: Air Pollution, in Manila. This region includes 16 countries, some of which are among the most densely populated in the world. Environmental needs of common interest to the region include:

(i)   Consideration of the general environmental pollution problems of the region.
(ii) Government activities to control them; that is, legislation for environmental protection.
(iii) National programmes for the effective implementation of the legislation.
(iv) Management organization—control regulations and the promulgation of acceptable and realistic environmental quality standards for various types of pollutants.
(v)   Standardization of sampling and testing techniques, of equipment and of analytical and reporting procedures for the monitoring of pollution and for testing at source.

(*vi*)   Provision of technical advisory services.

(*vii*) Training of technical personnel and the provision of a regional training centre.

(*viii*) Establishment of reference technical libraries and information services.

(*ix*)   Aspects of publicity and mass education.

(*x*)   Measures for implementing effective engineering control at source.

(*xi*)   Provision of locally manufactured pollution-control equipment.

(*xii*) Interrelationship of various types of pollution: air, water and land (soil).

(*xiii*) Promotion of joint research and development programmes on a regional basis.

(*xiv*) Allocation and control of fuels, with special reference to the use of 'polluting' fuels.

(*xv*)   Assessment of effects of pollutants on human and animal health, on materials and on vegetation—the organization of medical health surveys.

(*xvi*) Considerations of meteorological conditions and the selection of sites for industrial development in relation to urban developments.

(*xvii*) Promotion of regular meetings of personnel from related environmental protection organizations within the region, for regional cooperation and the exchange of knowledge and technology for the mutual benefit of the countries of the region.

The implementation of such measures is expensive and is therefore often low in the national priorities of developing countries: hence international assistance is needed.

Costs are involved, however, whether pollution is controlled or not, and the experience of developed countries indicates that while 'clean environment costs money; dirty environment costs more!' The economic costs of environmental pollution and its effects on human health, animal life, vegetation, materials, visibility, and so on, have been estimated in some of the developed countries to be many times more than the costs of controlling the problem. Moreover, the benefits of control cannot be assessed simply in terms of monetary return.

It is therefore not so much a question of 'Can we afford it?'—and we are all part of *one* world—but 'For how long can we neglect to take adequate action without suffering grave and irreversible consequences?'

Discussion

Dickinson: I am never sure whether to be horrified at the fact of pollution (as in Professor Kirov's examples) or to be cheered, as I was in my childhood in Lancashire, by the fact that when the black smoke reappeared, and the clogs started moving at 5.30 in the morning, people knew they were going to eat again. A static view of pollution is misleading in many ways. We must try to understand the dynamics of the situation. You can see many of the same things, as you have seen them in Taiwan, in mainland China, in Canton or in Shanghai, and the municipal authorities there tell you that they inherited this industry, that cleaning it up would cost a lot, and they recognize that there are always social costs which must be borne in order to change society. They see pollution as a problem but recognize that to spend scarce resources on solving it at this stage of development could be socially disadvantageous. They take the more long-term view of ensuring that the new industries that will eventually replace the old will produce less pollution.

In many developing countries where independence was achieved recently their older productive equipment will be disappearing in a relatively short time. In looking at the dynamics of the pollution situation we should consider that its elimination is an ongoing social aim rather than a short-term, and costly, technical problem. Even if we continue to expect growing standards of living, and if we control all pollution, there are ultimate limits to what the world can stand. In particular there is the thermal pollution limit which is the determining factor that will, in the last resort, limit economic growth of the kind we now pursue. No matter how clean we make industry, or how well we carry out all the elements of economic development, there is a finite limit to what we can do through industrialization. Ultimately this means accepting the redistribution of industrial potential and its benefits from those who have too much to those who have too little. Unless we can work for acceptance of this view our concept of the problem and its solution will remain unreal. I would like to see in this symposium some postulation of underlying hypotheses about a role that we could play in dealing with pollution in the context of the dynamics of world development. We can't say 'Stop. Let's get off this world and we will design a better one next week'. We have to start from where we are, but what we can do in the long term may best be achieved through a policy that neglects some of the more rapid, and costly, methods of eliminating pollution in the short term.

Kirov: The major problem at the moment is not to let new industries *develop* haphazardly, and produce all the pollution that we have to clean up afterwards. Much of it could be handled before it occurs by proper engineering. This is an area in which effective assistance could be given to developing countries, and which is not going to add to costs; you don't have to develop cities in such a way that all the pollution drains over the best areas of residential land; frequently, all that is needed is a little advice on meteorological conditions and how they operate, and therefore where factories should be located. If you look back to the 17th century when John Evelyn was writing here in London, he proposed things that we are not yet doing. He said that noxious industries should be taken out of the cities; we should separate the city areas from the industrial areas by green belts. We are not doing that yet.

Holland: It is essential to distinguish between the forms of pollution that can damage health and those that are harmful in the aesthetic sense. Professor Kirov tended to mix up these two forms of pollution and, in some of his examples, I doubt whether a real health hazard exists. This distinction is particularly important with environmental pollution. Before we indict it as a health hazard, there is need for far greater concentration on the evaluation of its effects on health.

Kirov: If you plot a graph of smoke density, with the increasing density of visible, apparent smoke you find an increasing proportion of associated invisible gases, carbon monoxide and carcinogenic hydrocarbons, emitted. Therefore it is not the smoke that we are worried about but the increasing proportion of the invisible hazardous gaseous components associated with the increasing density of smoke. Also, the smoke particles absorb sulphur and the combined effect of these two pollutants could have an important effect on health.

Holland: Although smoke and sulphur dioxide are clearly implicated in an increase in morbidity and mortality, we do not yet know whether one of these pollutants on its own is harmful, or whether they are only damaging in combination. To say that smoke particles absorb sulphur and the combined effects could have an important effect on health is too vague to be very meaningful. If doctors and engineers are to cooperate, it is essential that they both try to develop appropriate methods for measuring health effects as well as pollutant density.

Philip: I have become involved lately in Unesco's Man and Biosphere programme, which is concerned with the whole question of man's influence on the environment in which he and the rest of the organisms on this planet must live. I personally have had great difficulties in coming to grips with this huge question and in trying to get a perspective on it. One way which has seemed to me to be useful, and I am certainly not alone in this, is through looking at man's consumption of energy. It is not unreasonable to examine the implications of the approximation that pollution tends, in general, other things being equal, to be roughly proportional to energy consumption: and we may write the (tautological) equation,

density of energy consumption = (population density) × (energy consumption per head).

Population density is, I expect, outside our terms of reference, though I'm not sure it should be; but, in any case, I want to raise the question of per capita energy consumption. You will note that, other things being equal, the approximation I am examining implies that *the density of pollution is proportional to energy consumption per head.*

Ironically, we find that the ideal towards which many developing countries are struggling is the supposed material splendour of North America, complete with its pathologically high level of per capita energy consumption. In my view this poses problems not merely for the developing countries, but also for the developed ones. It seems to me essential that the developed countries make a deliberate effort to put a brake on their per capita energy consumption. (Let me make this quite clear: I urge this not on the usual and, I believe, less fundamental, ground that raw material and energy sources might be non-renewable, but from concern for man and the biosphere of which he is part.)

Specifically, the developed countries must consciously start to work out ways of life which are agreeable but don't need such idiotically high rates of energy consumption. This may well involve, among other things, some changes in the expectations of people. There is no real need to live in an air-conditioned house at 78 °F and go around naked in mid-winter, although that can be agreeable: many people in parts of the world other than North America have noticed that one can still survive in rooms at 45–50 °F, provided one has some clothes on! There is also the whole area of urban transport, of moving people around and of locating people. Work on these questions would represent only a start towards what I think should be a global strategy embracing both developing and developed countries: a deliberate effort to do something less ludicrous about energy and people. One highly desirable element in this (though it may not seem plausible to the developing countries until the developed countries display a certain amount of self-knowledge) would be a specific programme to bring into being low-energy industries, especially in the developing countries with their enormous resource of people. Professor Papanek's work on low-energy technologies is an admirable example of the concerned ingenuity needed to get such a movement under way.

All this may seem obvious. Indeed it is obvious and, in a sense, old hat. Yet the tacit assumptions of ever-increasing energy consumption and the extrapolation of recent trends in industrial growth remain all-pervading. Take, for example, the recent two-day Discussion on 'Energy in the 1980's' at the

Royal Society. This Discussion has now appeared in print and occupies 211 pages of the *Philosophical Transactions*[1]. Two hundred and ten and a half pages are devoted to discussion which accepts the present levels of energy consumption and extrapolates the trends of recent decades cheerfully and uncritically. One half page from Professor E. Eisner (p. 603), suggesting that we seek to reduce energy demands, evoked no response whatsoever. I hope this symposium will do better; though, at this stage, I am not sure.

Papanek: Let us not make the mistake here of being product-oriented; rather let us think about the process. Dr Philip mentioned the question of indoor comfort at certain temperatures, but his statistics make sense only if one thinks about 'a comfortably warm room' in terms of the end product. The energy expended for 'heating' in the UK is the second highest in the world, surpassed only in Norway. The *true* energy expended in the UK is really much greater than that in Norway since the amount of heat used in actually heating the average English home is between $\frac{1}{2}\%$ and 1%. Totally inefficient or non-existent insulation make the buildings chilly; in fact in some cases *all* the heat used in British homes heats the room only as an incidental by-pass while radiating out of the house. The energy cost could be lowered by truly fantastic-sounding figures (75–90%) if homes in the UK were insulated in a manner appropriate to the climate. In fact, the average house in England has insulation properties far below the standards considered minimal and mandatory for homes in the desert in Southern California, where temperatures vary between 65 and 115 °F.

Philip: Of course we must use what we know to reduce energy consumption; and the insulation of buildings is an excellent example. But my point was that we must go further and look searchingly at prevalent fashions in human expectations about comfort, solitary travel, and so forth.

Porter: It might be helpful if we focus specifically on the way in which health hazards change with different stages of development or industrialization. Although industrialization carries with it side-effects and pollution hazards, I think most people would agree that industrialized Britain in 1974 *is* a much healthier place, on all the usual indicators of health, than less-industrialized Britain was 100 or 200 years ago. In the case of the poor countries, it is by no means self-evident that, for example in South-East Asia or India, the health situation in unindustrialized villages is 'better', in some sense, than the health situation in moderately sized cities. In any event, it would be useful to examine the evidence. Of course, when cities grow very large—like Calcutta, for example—a different order of health hazards are created and different ways of dealing with them have to be devised. However, it would be reasonable to assume that public health and preventive medicine are more easily brought to people if they are grouped in medium-sized communities (say, cities of upwards of 100 000) rather than scattered over wide areas. We should not lose sight of the benefits that industrialization can bring, including a greater production of goods and services (which *is* surely desirable), through a preoccupation with the second-order effects. I do not believe that people in developing countries, and certainly very poor people, aspire to the standard of living of the US. I do not think that the 40% of the Indian population living on one rupee a day aspire to such standards; but they doubtless do want to be in a position to produce sufficient food for themselves and to have an economic system that will provide them with adequate clothing, better housing, and so on, and this involves increased energy consumption. It may take one up from say 1/8 ton to two tons a year, and this will involve a new order of health problems, but I do not think that the health problems associated with that change will be of the same order as the health problems associated with poverty on the scale existing now all over the developing world. It is easy for those of us living in a comparatively affluent society to talk about the horrors of industrialization but many people in poor countries would gladly accept the miseries of *our* industrial society in exchange for the miseries they get with low energy consumption.

Ramalingaswami: The romance of rural life really is no longer there. To give one example: the incidence of tuberculosis in the rural population of India is almost identical with that in the cities, something like 1–2%, so you don't find the difference that you might expect. What is happening in the garb of urbanization is really the 'ruralization' of cities; you are creating in cities like Calcutta an environmental arena that is no different from a scattered but nevertheless clustered group of houses in a rural setting.

Kirov: When we talk about energy consumption we should make a distinction between standards of living and the quality of life. In the developing countries the two rise together, so that such countries see industrialization as something that will provide them with better health, jobs, housing, food, education, and opportunities through life. But the developed countries can increase their gross national product per capita at a higher rate because of their more stable population, and therefore they are just adding to their material standards but the quality of life does not necessarily increase. We should be talking about 20 or 30 years from now; by the year 2000, the world population could stabilize, if action is taken *now*, at about 7000 million people. If we continue to increase the consumption of energy in the West we are not improving the quality of life but we are drawing on resources which are exhaustible. The question is not whether poorer countries should develop, but to what extent should the developed countries de-escalate their own developments in order to share out more evenly the finite resources of the world.

Ashby: Dr White warned us earlier (p. 11) that we have to be careful about extrapolating experience from industrial countries to other kinds of countries. We have learnt this in education, where we in Britain have exported universities to places like Africa in the sort of way we have exported motor cars. Just as Chevrolet cars exported to Lagos still have a de-frosting device switched on from the dashboard, so the curricula we exported carried the educational equivalents of de-frosting devices. We had to learn how to adapt our indigenous educational system to African needs. But there are experiences we can legitimately pick out as being valuable for export; for example, the realization that medical services would be much better *not* fragmented (e.g. between domiciliary practice and industrial practice) as they are in the UK. This is something that WHO is putting into its blueprint, and it seems to be a valuable point. A further useful contribution which the UK and other European countries can offer, suggested by Dr Gilson (p. 27), is to make our health records available. Unlike those of most developing countries, our health records are now old enough for us to begin to draw statistical conclusions about one of the very perplexing problems in occupational health and environmental health, namely the long-term effects on health of low concentrations of substances. Until you have kept records for many years you can't begin to discover whether or not there are such effects.

Reference

1. Energy in the 1980's (1974) *Philosophical Transactions of the Royal Society of London, Series A 276*, 405-615

Some environmental health problems associated with industrial development in Ghana

L. K. A. DERBAN

> *The most valuable capital of the State and of Society is man, and to protect him is not merely the dictate of humanitarian sentiment but a duty imposed by self-interest on every community.*
>
> PRINCE RUDOLF

It is generally agreed that rational industrialization can help to accelerate socioeconomic development in a country and that every sector of the economy has a health component of such importance that it cannot be disregarded in any major development programme. Man is undeniably an indispensable factor in production, and his total environment plays a dominant part in determining the level of his physical and mental health and his social well-being.

In Ghana, as in all other developing countries, we can group problems of the human environment into two categories:

(1) Those that are the result of poverty and lack of development.
(2) Those that are the result of the development process itself.

Although in this paper I shall mainly discuss the environmental health problems of industrial development, it is worth remembering that in Ghana the environmental problems are predominantly the basic ones:

(1) Inadequate supply of sufficient drinking water.
(2) Poor or non-existent waste disposal systems for human excreta and refuse.
(3) Undernutrition and malnutrition.
(4) Inadequate housing.
(5) Abundant disease vectors (insects and higher animals).

Much of the rapid industrialization in Ghana followed Independence in 1957. There is overwhelming evidence that this rapid economic development has in some cases led to undesirable environmental consequences—the deterioration of natural resources, pollution, problems of resettlement, and many health problems—thus negating, to a certain extent, the presumed aim of national development, namely the welfare of man.

Rapid industrialization and its environmental health problems have therefore to be viewed against the background of the general health problems of the country—the tremendous problems posed by the natural demographic expansion, the high rate of mortality, the high prevalence of communicable diseases, undernutrition and malnutrition, inadequate health manpower and facilities, illiteracy and a lack of financial resources.

GENERAL HEALTH PROBLEMS OF GHANA

The salient points are as follows. The population is 8.6 million by the 1970 census.[1] Twenty per cent of the people are under five years of age and 45% are under 15 years of age and, therefore, not really contributors to the general economy.

The rate of population growth is between 2.7% and 3.3% per year. It is estimated that at such a rate of increase the population will double itself in about 30 years. This rapid population growth can jeopardize national aspirations for economic and social development and can adversely affect the welfare of families and the health of individuals.

Health statistics

From the Registrar General's statistics, the birth rate is 47 per thousand inhabitants. The crude death rate is 22 per thousand. The maternal mortality rate is 17 per thousand live births and the infant mortality is 110 per thousand live births. These figures are averages and they hide very large fluctuations between some of the big towns and rural areas, as was shown in a recent survey in which the maternal mortality rate in Accra was found to be six per thousand live births while in the rural areas it was 35. Similarly, the infant mortality rate in Accra was 38 per thousand live births, and in rural areas, 167.

Morbidity

Of all the people who die, almost one-third die from communicable diseases. Malaria, tuberculosis, gastrointestinal infections, malnutrition, schistosomiasis and onchocerciasis, though preventable or curable, are still widespread causes of sickness, disability and premature death. There are still areas where worm infections—particularly roundworms, hookworms and guinea worms—are more or less universal and where leprosy is not uncommon.

Throughout the country there is a need for adequate environmental sanitation. Adequate and dependable water supplies have reached only a fraction of the population. In some areas, the population use the same small river or stream for all their daily water requirements. They wash in it, bathe in it, and take it for cooking purposes. This results in a high incidence of parasitic and bacterial infections, particularly enteric fevers, dysentery and cholera. Progress in environmental sanitation has been slow, due mainly to lack of properly organized community efforts and lack of financial resources.

There are also serious food and nutritional problems. The main causes are low agricultural production, storage difficulties, inadequate marketing facilities, and poor selection and utilization of the available food. Drought has recently become a very important factor in the northern zone of the country.

The effects of poor diet on socioeconomic development are undeniable, though difficult to measure or isolate. Chronic diseases when combined with malnutrition are known to have a cumulative effect, leading to severe disability which interferes with the individual's capacity to work and lowers his productivity and earnings.

In children, protein-calorie (i.e. protein energy) malnutrition is a major problem. Poverty and ignorance are probably the chief causes. In Ghana, many of the dietary problems are in fact seasonal in nature, and have therefore to be viewed from the practical point of view and carefully related to prevailing agricultural standards, as is being emphasized by the current 'operation feed yourself' programme, with some measure of success.

The main orientation and development of the health services in the country has tended to concentrate on curative rather than on preventive services and the institutions of those services have been concentrated in towns rather than in rural areas. Hospital care programmes have tended to be expensive. The country is short of all categories of health workers.

Ghanaian society is now increasingly being led to expect a great deal more from medical science than before. The Government and the medical profession are therefore being challenged to look critically at the health care system, which must provide health care to most people with the available limited resources in ways that will yield the greatest benefit.

There is a growing awareness in Ghana of the importance of the preventive aspects of the health services and local health training institutions are now providing adequate training and experience that will enable health personnel to cope with community as well as individual health problems.

INDUSTRIALIZATION IN GHANA

Although Ghana's economy is basically agricultural, much emphasis has been put on industrialization since Independence. Ghana today is committed, as a national policy, to the systematic assessment and exploitation of her natural resources. The goals are: an improved economy, a favourable balance of trade, self-reliance and self-sufficiency in the production of raw materials and foodstuffs, an increase in commerce and trade for its citizens, and an improvement of social services—especially education, communications and health care.

Before the Second World War, industries in Ghana were limited to the semi-processing of agricultural products needed in Europe. The only truly indigenous industries were of African artisans working in iron, leather, copper, gold, clay and fibre. There were virtually no manufacturing industries apart from these. More recently, however, there has been a rapid growth of industries. The number of manufacturing industries increased from 167 in 1962 to 356 in 1969. Most of these industries are small-sized establishments providing the primary occupation for a considerable number of people.

Apart from the small-scale traditional industrial enterprises scattered all over the country, several pioneer industries have been set up, particularly in the modern industrial complexes that have come into being in the Accra-Tema area, the Sekondi-Takoradi area, and the Kumasi area.

Mining (gold, diamonds, bauxite and manganese) has become a major industry in Ghana, second to agriculture.

The giant Volta River Project, officially inaugurated in January 1966, aims primarily at generating electric power for the processing of Ghana's bauxite and at feeding the electric generating network supplying many areas in Ghana.

HEALTH HAZARDS TO THE COMMUNITY FROM INDUSTRIES

The rapid industrial development in Ghana has had a serious impact on the quality of the human environment. Some of the major factors involved are urbanization and migration; the industrial pollution of air, water and soil; the use of pesticides; and river basin development and resettlement. These will be considered in turn.

Urbanization and migration

In Ghana most towns began to develop only with the arrival of territorial administrations and the interrelated penetration of commerce and communications. Small market centres and ports have, with increasing urbanization in recent years, become towns (see Table 1). Since Independence in 1957, urban growth, particularly in the regional capitals representing the new development areas, has been accelerated by the encouragement of industry and commerce,

TABLE 1

Urban population growth in Ghana: the percentage of the population in towns with more than 5000 inhabitants

Year	% of population in towns with more than 5000 people
1921	6.9%
1931	9.5%
1948	13.4%
1960	23.1%
1970	29.6%

Source: Population Census of Ghana[1].

the setting up of institutions such as universities and secondary schools, and the increase in administrative positions.

It has been recognized that a supply of labour amenable to supervision and responsive to economic incentives is a prerequisite for sustained industrial growth. Such a labour force is beginning to develop in Ghana, although migrant labour is quite common[2].

Much of this urban growth has been possible only because of migration from the rural areas, hence the above-average annual rate of increase in the populations of the towns and cities (see Table 2). This rapid growth of populations in the urban areas has posed serious environmental health problems.

In a recent survey, the main reasons given by people who migrated from rural to urban areas were:

(i) To look for work.
(ii) To seek education.

TABLE 2

Rates of growth of the urban areas in Ghana (The average annual birth rate is 2.0-3.0%)

Town or city	Number of inhabitants 1960	1970	% increase 1960-1970	Annual rate of increase
Accra	337 828	564 194	67.01	6.1
Kumasi	180 642	260 286	44.09	4.1
Sekondi-Takoradi	75 450	91 874	21.77	2.0
Tamale	40 443	83 653	106.84	9.7
Cape Coast	41 230	51 653	25.28	2.3
Koforidua	34 856	46 235	32.65	3.0
Ho	14 519	24 196	66.65	6.1
Sunyani	12 160	23 780	95.56	8.7
Bolgatanga	5 500	18 896	243.56	22.1

(*iii*) To seek environmental change and the enjoyment of what they regard
as the better urban life.

Both men and women migrate. The migrants work in a range of unskilled
occupations on construction works, in the mines, and in manufacturing
industries. People moving from the rural areas to towns usually arrive with
severe handicaps, such as lack of education or of training for any job. They
are also unable to adjust emotionally and are misinformed about town life
generally. They find themselves on the fringes of the town society, both
physically and socially. This results in the growth of slums and shanty towns
around the big industrial areas with their accompanying serious environmental
health problems, particularly of overcrowding, a high incidence of disease,
and sociocultural disintegration, which lay the foundation for behavioural
problems such as delinquency, crime, prostitution and alcoholism.

A recent survey in one of the gold-mining areas showed a high incidence of
tuberculosis in the immigrants, a result of the presence of a large number of
resident silico-tuberculosis patients (retired miners) living in bad conditions in
the shanty towns which encourage the spread of this disease.

Dr T. A. Lambo has noted that the biggest problems of migrant labour in
Africa are malnutrition, venereal disease, and crippling neurosis. Being
unsettled, the migrants not only pose a problem of spreading communicable
diseases from place to place but also of hindering detection, treatment and the
follow-up programmes necessary for control. A recent outbreak of smallpox
in the Accra-Tema area was traced to a migrant who had just arrived, in-
cubating the disease. Migrant fishing communities suffering from urinary
schistosomiasis are a major factor in the spread of the disease in villages along
the shores of the Volta Lake, which were previously free from the disease.

Experience has shown that any health programme designed to reach such a
group effectively must be multidisciplinary in character and should include such
activities as mass-screening procedures, treatment, horizontal health surveys,
food and nutrition surveys, social welfare and community development, and
health education. The Kotobabi polyclinic project and the Nima community
development project, both in the suburbs of Accra, and the Akosombo industrial community health programme set up by the Volta River Authority,
are serious attempts to find effective ways of reaching such a group of migrant
labourers and their families. The important feature of these programmes is the
use they make of paramedical personnel to provide primary patient care.

Of the various categories of migrants, the elementary school leaver group is
considered to cause the greatest social and economic problems. In order to
reduce the migration of this group from rural to urban areas the development

of more rural industries and settlement farms is seriously being considered. The Development Banks and the Regional Development Corporations are expected to play a more positive role in systematic rural agricultural financing than before.

Industrial pollution of the environment

An epidemic of arsenic poisoning occurred in a gold-mining community in Ghana[3]. Investigations revealed gross contamination of the atmosphere, soil, water and vegetation by arsenic discharged into the air during extraction processes at the gold mine. The contamination with arsenic was found in the surrounding area up to 40 miles away. Rainwater collected in the area for drinking contained up to six parts per million of arsenic and creek water into which the mine wastes were discharged contained up to eight parts per million. Broad plantain leaves in the area contained up to 650 parts per million and the dry vegetation around a great deal more.

Poisoning was found to be due to skin contact with arsenic dust, drinking of water containing arsenic, or inhalation of arsenic dust in the atmosphere. The main clinical features were conjunctivitis, chronic lesions with skin mottling and hyperpigmentation, bronchitis and gastrointestinal disturbances. Hair and urine samples from affected people showed up to 500 parts per million and two parts per million respectively, indicating a high intake of arsenic.

Such environmental pollution can be prevented by constant supervision, proper occupational health and environmental control programmes, health education and legislation. The newly created Environmental Protection Council in Ghana is an attempt by the Government to provide machinery for preventing such environmental problems.

Agriculture and pesticides

Agriculture is the mainstay of Ghana's economy. Consequently it should be a highly efficient, productive and safe occupation. But the rapid increase in both the amount and number of pesticides available in Ghana for use in agriculture and public health has caused general concern about the risks to public health from modern chemical pesticides in foodstuffs and in the environment. Pesticides become environmental pollutants if they are transferred from the area of intended application or if they persist in the environment longer than necessary.

The multiplicity of pesticides designed for specific purposes in the hands of people who may not be aware of their toxicity has led to trouble. For instance, consumption of a foodstuff 'tuo-soffi' which was contaminated by an insecticide resulted in ten cases of poisoning and three deaths. The food was made up of cornmeal mixed with a small amount of concentrated (25%) gammaxene, which has the same appearance and can be mistaken for cassava meal.

Recently, a total of 144 cases of alkylmercury poisoning with 20 deaths were reported in rural southern Ghana. Their ages ranged from $1\frac{1}{2}$ to 74 years[4]. Out of ignorance, the patients had eaten maize which was dressed with ethyl mercuric chloride and was intended for sowing. In this outbreak, those involved were aware of the poisonous nature of the pesticide but were under the false impression that thorough washing of the dressed grain with warm water would remove all the poison. What makes the situation in Ghana perhaps unique is that this erroneous impression was enforced by past experience in removing enough DDT from maize to avoid any clinical effects. Practically an entire village was affected, because the village was regarded as one family and people ate freely at one another's table.

Agricultural pollution calls for close coordination with the health services in order to ensure high agricultural productivity without health hazards to people and livestock. At present the cultural and educational background necessary for the effective introduction of safety precautions is lacking. The nature of agricultural work makes control difficult or impossible. Education, training and medical surveillance are difficult to organize, especially in scattered rural communities whose educational standards are often low. In these circumstances, strict control of the importing of extremely toxic agricultural chemical compounds may be an important measure in the effective control of pesticides in the country.

The enormous problems that can arise out of the improper use of chemical pesticides have led to the urgent search for an alternative to chemicals in an improved pest control system. In Ghana, the biological control of the oil palm leaf miner beetle (*Coelaenomenodeca edaeidis*) by other insects has been used for the past few years with good results. The egg and larval parasites used have had such a pronounced effect on the population dynamics of the host pest that they have eliminated the use of chemicals. This is particularly important since the use of chemical pesticides in the oil palm plantations may lead to problems with pesticide residues in the palm oil, which is used for cooking.

Pigs have been used to eradicate snakes in the moist undergrowths in oil palm and sugarcane plantations.

Biological control has its problems. For its successful application a critical knowledge is required of the relationship between the biological control agents, the target organism, and the other members of the ecosystem. There is also the need for coordination between the scientist in the laboratory and the field operators.

Integrated pest control has received serious consideration by FAO's expert panel and other scientists as an essential approach to solving pest problems. This system of pest management involves the use of possible alternative methods of control, namely biological control, plant resistance, crop manipulation, physical and chemical agents, and genetic and biological techniques. This approach requires much planning and research if successful integrated pest control programmes are to be set up in a developing country.

THE VOLTA RIVER BASIN DEVELOPMENT

Mainly in order to diversify the economy of Ghana by changing the commodity structure of agriculture and industry, the Government paid serious attention to the development of Ghana's hydro-electric power and bauxite potential in an aluminium industry in 1959. This led to the construction of the Akosombo Dam (1961–1964), the generation of the first power and the start of production by an aluminium smelter using imported alumina in 1966.

The building of the dam on the Volta River and the consequent formation of the new Volta Lake (Fig. 1) with a surface area of 3275 square miles (3.6% of the surface of Ghana) created a number of development possibilities in fisheries, agriculture, transport, wildlife and tourism. The lake also changed the existing physical, biological and socioeconomic environment of the people and the patterns of disease, and created conditions in which the risks of explosive outbreaks of infections could be high[5,6].

The Volta River Authority, assisted by the UN Development Programme, started research into the public health situation and resettlement of the people displaced by the Volta Lake and also research on fisheries and hydrobiology. Specifically it concentrated on:

(i) The public health problems of waterborne diseases associated with the lake and the means of their control.

(ii) New systems of agriculture and other incentives for the resettled people.

(iii) The limnology and fish biology of the lake and the means of exploiting the fish stocks.

Resettlement problems

The human problem of resettlement was by far the most serious impact of the Volta River project[7]. A census-type of social survey made before the resettlement showed that approximately 80 000 people, or 1% of the population,

58 L. K. A. DERBAN

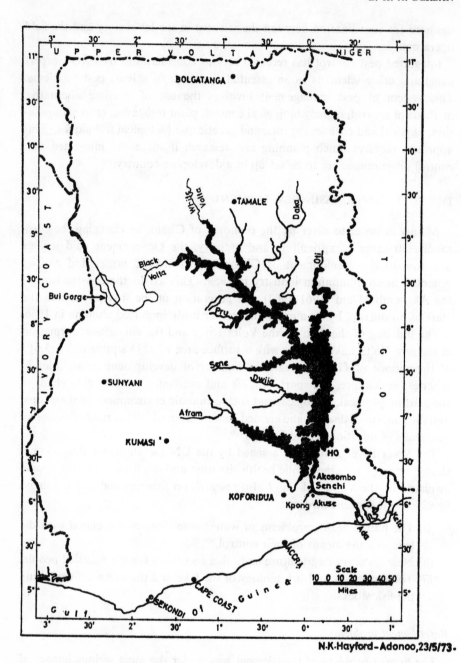

FIG. 1. Map of Ghana, showing the Volta Lake.

lived in the area and therefore had to be resettled. About 85% of the people (67 500) were to be settled in 52 resettlement sites scattered around the lake (see Fig. 2). Some 12 500 people (15%) chose to resettle themselves. The people who were resettled came from four regions of the country and had lived in the river basin for many years. A total of 739 villages were destroyed. About 14 657 households were disrupted; 12 799 households with 173 domestic animals including 36 cattle and 195 birds had to be moved. The people were mostly subsistence farmers. Only 2% of them were river fishermen.

The main resettlement objectives of the Volta River Authority were:

(1) To provide dwelling, work and recreation places for the settlers.
(2) To offer the settlers an opportunity for productive work.
(3) To improve the physical appearance of their surrounding landscape.
(4) To help the settlers to develop a community spirit.

The facilities provided included houses, offices, schools, playgrounds, markets, water supplies, streets, latrines and farms.

Socioeconomic problems

One of the major problems was the organization of the settlements into institutions with budgets and personnel to make them work. The challenge was therefore to support the settlers so that they could develop their farms and build their towns into living and orderly communities which satisfied their needs for health, safety and well-being.

Houses were provided, but the settlers had to make them into homes. The resettlements were bleak and featureless with no familiar market days for buying, selling and social contact. The settlers had exchanged a place of comfort for a place of insecurity. This initial stage was a period of social and economic constraint and stress. It took a long time before fishing and farming could be brought to a reasonable efficiency. It was therefore necessary to supply food, through the World Food Programme.

One of the most serious problems which the Volta River Authority had to face during the early years of resettlement was that of administration[8]. The Volta River Authority, set up primarily tor generate electric power, found itself not fully equipped to handle the administrative problems of the resettlement. Town Managers were created to manage the affairs of resettlement through Town Development Committees. This arrangement made it very difficult to integrate the statuses and roles of the different traditional authorities brought together in the exercise. The social cohesion and order were seriously affected.

Lack of community life and the slow improvement in the physical and

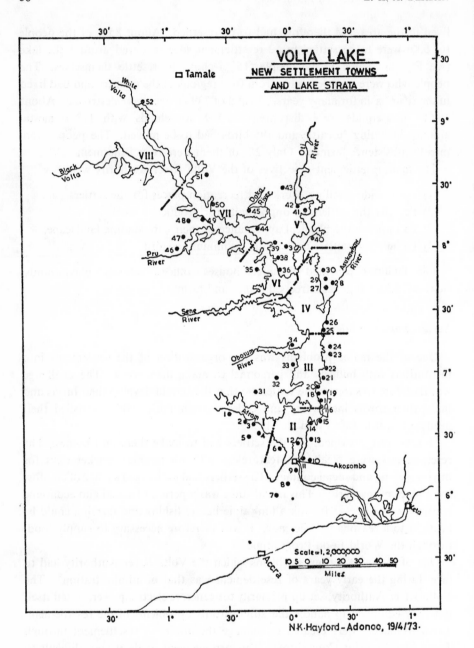

FIG. 2. Map of the Volta Lake, showing the new settlement towns and lake strata. Key opposite.

economic environment led to the drift out of the resettlement towns of some of the able-bodied people, leaving behind the very young and the old and infirm. Thus in 1968, 60% of the original settlers had moved out, a trend which has recently been reversed by a positive and more effective approach to land acquisition and distribution.

The transfer of responsibility to the local authorities and Technical Departments of the Government had its initial problems, but has improved the situation.

Environmental sanitation

Ignorance, apathy, and local customs and habits led to marked indifference to public health problems in the settlements. The communal latrines provided (the aqua-privy variety) soon ceased to function as a result of lack of proper use and maintenance. Frequent breakdowns of the sewage collection and disposal system led to indiscriminate dumping of refuse and defaecation.

Pipe-water systems operated by diesel pumps soon failed. The pumps broke down and there were no funds for fuel. The public water stand-pipes were not properly looked after and were soon in need of repair. With the breakdown of the water supply and sewage disposal in some settlement areas, conditions became favourable for the possible increase of waterborne diseases such as typhoid fever, dysentery and other diarrhoeal diseases, parasitic diseases such as hookworm diseases, and insect-borne diseases.

Local councils had great difficulty in maintaining these misused health

←

KEY

1. New Oworobong	14. Tonkor/Kaira	27. Kantanka	40. Dumbai
2. Kwahu Amanfrom	15. Todome	28. Akroso Amanfrom	41. Kitare
3. Dedeso Wireko	16. Tsohor	29. Adonkwanta	42. Bladjae
4. Dominase	17. Botoku	30. Tokroano	43. Kpandae
5. Onuku	18. Wusuta	31. Forifori	44. Grube
6. Anyaboni	19. Vakpo Dunyo	32. Mem Chemte	45. Gulubi
7. Adukrom	20. Savalu	33. Amankwakrom	46. Prang
8. Somanya	21. Danyigba	34. Ntoaboma	47. Labun
9. Senchi	22. Fesi	35. Kajaj	48. Buma
10. Apequsu	23. Tepo	36. Kete Krachi	49. Yeji
11. Mpakadam	24. Wurupong	37. Ntewusa	50. Makongo
12. New Ajena	25. Bowri Odumasi	38. Osramani	51. Bawu
13. Nkwakubew	26. Tapa Abotoase	39. Ohiamankyene	52. Yapei

facilities. Deep pit latrines were found to be more suitable and pipe-water systems operated by hand pumps gave satisfactory results.

An intensive health education programme had to be launched to help people who were then facing conditions which required a higher standard of health than they were used to.

Mental health

The psychological trauma caused by the sudden removal of the settlers from their familiar surroundings to a strange environment made their cooperation in the move difficult. The settlers needed a lot of encouragement and support to raise their economic status, in order to boost their morale.

The experiences of the Volta Resettlement in Ghana have been embodied in a symposium report[7].

HEALTH PROBLEMS ASSOCIATED WITH THE FORMATION OF THE LAKE

Right from the start it was realized that the Volta Lake would have a considerable impact on public health. There was therefore a need for a continuous study of the health of the population in the neighbourhood of the lake, with emphasis on schistosomiasis, onchocerciasis, trypanosomiasis and malaria[9]. These studies were done through the public health section of the Volta Lake Research and Development Project being assisted by the UN Development Programme. Its immediate objective was the control of the major parasitic diseases, as an essential step for the development of the economic potential.

Schistosomiasis

Schistosomiasis (bilharzia) is a snail-borne infection which might be expected in water development schemes. An epidemiological survey made before the lake was formed, in 1960–1961, showed that its endemicity was low along the Volta River. The prevalence in school children was 5%[11]. Surveys in 1964–1967, after construction of the dam, showed a 90% rate in school children with a ratio of two boys to one girl. The prevalence of urinary schistosomiasis in the Volta Dam area varies considerably according to locality and surveys have revealed a gradual rise in the incidence of the disease where previously the infection rates were moderate or nil.

The increase in the disease in certain localities after the lake's formation has been found to be due to (a) a biological explosion of aquatic weeds and snails, and (*b*) the migration into the area of fishing communities already suffering from urinary schistosomiasis. The aquatic weeds which are important as the habitat of the snail vector are *Ceratophyllum*, *Alternanthera*, *Spirodela* and *Pistia*. The snail vector is especially abundant in beds of the dominant submerged plant *Ceratophyllum*[11].

The snail *Bulinus truncatus rohlfsi* is the commonest and most widely distributed in the lake and can survive at a depth of 4.57 metres. *Bulinus globosus* is also an important schistosome host in Ghana but its distribution in the lake is restricted.

Transmission occurs in the lake itself. Exposure to infestation is high, especially for fishermen who dive to get fish traps, as well as for people, particularly children, who draw water from the lake or bathe in it.

It has proved difficult to control the snail vector by eliminating the aquatic weeds. The effective herbicides have the undesirable side-effect of contaminating drawdown soil and inhibiting the growth of some crops, particularly tobacco and tomatoes. Mechanized clearing requires continuous labour to be successful and is impracticable because of the large areas involved.

Where the disease is prevalent but transmission is known to have ceased, mass clinical treatment is undertaken.

The problem of urinary schistosomiasis must be seen as a disease complex which embraces both the lake and the Volta delta. The migratory habits of the fishermen ensure the spread of the disease from endemic areas to other areas. The present situation of the disease in the Volta Lake cannot be viewed with optimism. Re-surveys of some localities have shown an increased prevalence which points rather to a deteriorating situation, with the disease increasing in the areas where infection rates were previously found to be low.

It is realized that to prevent continuing transmission of the disease, a long-term education programme, combined with effective sanitary measures, including an efficient disposal system for excreta, a safe water supply and adequate bathing and washing facilities, is necessary.

Onchocerciasis (river blindness)

This disease is carried by the blackfly, *Simulium damnosum*. Breeding is limited to well-oxygenated water—rapidly flowing streams and rivers[10]. The fly and disease were previously widespread along the Volta River. When the lake was formed many of the major breeding sites in the river were eliminated, but the fast flow below the dam enhanced the breeding possibilities at the rapids there. The disease, therefore, has not been wiped out with the eradication of the fly by the formation of the lake. In some areas below the dam, and also near the rapid streams, prevalence rates among all people over 15 years of age are as high as 90%, and infection has been found in children as young as two years old; nodules have been found in four-year-old children. Ocular complications have been detected.

Since 1962 control by means of chemicals has been directed against the aquatic stages of the fly below the dam. Periodic spilling through the sluice gates of the dam, intended to dislodge the larvae, is a useful adjunct to the chemical control but has not been used in recent years because of the low rainfall. Re-infestation from several small streams entering the Volta River below the dam is considerable.

The proposed secondary dam to be constructed below the Akosombo Dam—the Kpong project—will reduce the problem of onchocerciasis transmission in the immediate vicinity but will increase the problem of schistosomiasis.

A local onchocerciasis control operation is desirable and urgently needed, but total eradication by modern techniques and pesticides can only be achieved through a comprehensive and imaginative onchocerciasis control programme in the entire Volta River Basin area in West Africa. This inter-regional control programme has been planned and is a combined effort of the seven West African countries—Ghana, Togo, Niger, Mali, Upper Volta, the Ivory Coast and Dahomey—and the Food and Agriculture Organization, the World Health Organization, the International Bank for Reconstruction and Development (the World Bank) and the UN Development Project. It started in March 1974.

Trypanosomiasis (African sleeping sickness)

African sleeping sickness is carried by the tsetse fly (*Glossina palpalis*), its principal vector. The fly is associated with the lakeside and riverside, more especially in the light forest fringing the edge of the water.

The formation of the lake has been beneficial in that it drowned large areas of forest which once harboured tsetse flies. The prevalence of the disease in the river basin is low in spite of the wide distribution of the flies. In 1971, six cases of sleeping sickness were diagnosed and treated at the health centres. In 1972 and 1973, only two cases were reported.

With the vegetation pattern around the lake changing and evolving during the years, and population movements and river transportation now on the increase, attention is being paid to the probable development of new endemic foci and the appearance of clinical cases of the disease.

Mosquitoes and disease

Mosquito surveys have been going on since 1971, with the following aims:

(*i*) To determine the species breeding in the lake.
(*ii*) To determine the species associated with man.
(*iii*) To determine their role in the transmission of malaria, filariasis, and any other mosquito-borne diseases.

Malaria

The principal vectors of malaria in this region are *Anopheles gambiae, A. funestus, A. nili* and *A. hargreaves*. Malaria is hyper-endemic in Ghana and there is no reason to suppose that the epidemiology of the disease has changed in the region since the formation of the lake.

Bancroftian filariasis

The vectors of this disease in rural Ghana are *A. gambiae* and *A. funestus*. Very few overt cases of the disease have been found in the Volta basin. *Mansonia africanus* has been found associated with the aquatic plant *Pistia*, but there is no evidence of this mosquito being a vector of the disease.

Mosquito-borne viral infections (yellow fever and dengue)

The most important of the arthropod-borne viral infections that have received attention are yellow fever and dengue. The vector of these diseases is *Aedes aegypti* which breeds in small collections of water in tins, coconut shells and discarded car tyres. The breeding and distribution of this mosquito was encouraged during the early part of the resettlement programme by the breakdown of the refuse-collecting system and the water supply pumps in the resettlement villages, which meant that water had to be stored in jars and drums. The problem was therefore associated with resettlement and was an indirect effect of the formation of the lake. The disease has been successfully controlled by mass inoculation and by an attack on the breeding sites.

The public health section of the Volta Lake Research and Development Project continues to update health data relating to the lake, to evaluate and keep under surveillance the major health problems, to make field investigations into incidence and to forecast disease trends. It makes recommendations on health facilities and plans, and carries out and evaluates vector control programmes in cooperation with the Ministry of Health.

CONCLUSION

It is generally agreed that all developing countries must modernize the industrial sector of their economies and reinforce the base for a self-sustaining economy. It is, however, important to industrialize in the best interests of the people, the environment, and the totality of the economy. The concept of industrialization should be broadened to include not only factories for manufacturing processes but also facilities for people's educational, recreational, social and health needs—hence the need for environmentally oriented industrial planning.

Since one of the key indicators of deleterious environmental influences is the status of human health itself, there is the need to develop a system of integrated surveillance and monitoring of human health and well-being in relation to environmental factors.

The responsibility for the rational management and use of the resources of a country and for the conservation of the environment rests on the government. Some countries, including Ghana, have set up a multidisciplinary national Environmental Protection Council to be responsible for the environmental aspects of development and for research programmes associated with the rational use of natural resources. Because of the complex interaction between natural and social sciences that is needed if one is to approach the problems of economic development, it is necessary to give special consideration to the organizational aspects of multidisciplinary studies.

The success of any environmentally oriented industrial programme lies in the total support and collaboration of policy makers, industrialists, natural and social scientists, and the general public. The importance of education and training in environmental questions at all levels therefore cannot be over-emphasized if citizens are to be informed, educated and motivated to use their land and natural resources properly. We must encourage activities designed to bring together the various groups to discuss and study all aspects of the impact of economic development on the total environment. To quote Dr Johnson: 'To preserve health is a moral and religious duty, for health is the basis of all social virtues—we can no longer be useful when not well'.

Discussion

Bridger: Dr Derban, you described the multidisciplinary approach to the Volta resettlement scheme but this apparently didn't include people familiar with the type of processes that go on in groups and in organizations. By this I mean people interested in cross-cultural development who understand the dynamics involved. I am thinking of work done on the resettlement of prisoners of war after 1945, and recent work on the re-location of civil servants in the UK[12-14]. Such work is concerned not only with the specific situations but just as much with the *processes* going on in resettlement, in re-location and in reorganization[15]; not least, the process of planning itself has to be considered as a dynamic, not just as a sequential procedure.

Mars: I would like to explore these questions of dynamics and process a little further. It seems to me that there may well be differences between identifying the needs of the people concerned as they are seen by specialist surveyors and identifying the needs of people as they perceive themselves, which involves a different way of working. The former is now extensively carried out and its justification has reached the level of a conventional wisdom. For the latter, however, you need, as an innovator, to work through communities and you need to have people working with you who are resident in these communities both before and after any transition. This is not the only way, but I think it one of the best ways by which one can begin to understand social processes and their dynamics in the type of community we are discussing.

Dr Derban said that 60% of the people were leaving the resettlements and that a high proportion of these were the able-bodied men. But why were they leaving? What was not provided in the new situations that would have made them want to stay? I would suggest that it is this type of question that can best be examined through internal community studies. In my paper (pp. 219–228) I shall be putting forward the idea of 'barefoot' sociologists—or what might better be called 'barefoot anthropologists'. Like Chinese barefoot doctors, these would also be auxiliaries and they would be used to attempt to link social reality to social planning. I would see them as locally based, locally resident and locally involved but able to work to and through a fully trained coordinating professional who could thereby monitor up to, say, ten communities.

You also talked, Dr Derban, about community medicine. Have you seen Frankenberg and Leeson's article[16] on the suggestion of a barefoot doctor service for Zambia? They point out that nearly all the country's medical resources are concentrated in the capital but that if these were distributed in the Chinese pattern, it could provide an auxiliary medical service for every community in the country. The cost of both anthropological and medical auxiliary services would be relatively small, and I see them as complementary— perhaps with both functions linked to the same role. I would suggest, however, that what one needs to get away from is the 'wise man' from the city (whether planner, sociologist or physician) who goes out to the villages, deduces what their needs are from the standpoint of his discipline's concern and techniques, and then derives or amends policy from this standpoint and experience.

Derban: The disciplinary approach to the settlement scheme I described, in fact, included Community Development Assistants who were carefully selected and trained. They were then locally based and locally resident, and they helped to explain and sell the Volta River Project to the people and persuaded them to accept evacuation happily. In the settlement towns, the Community Development Assistants took on other functions such as adult education, care of the blind and the imparting of domestic skills to the women.

The resettlement programme was intended to be carried out in logical phases but the urgency of the operation and other factors meant that all aspects of the programme went on simultaneously, thus creating a dynamic situation of constant change and flux. The agricultural programme which was so vital for the ultimate viability of the resettlement was also beset with difficulties from the start. It was this combination of factors that led to the lack of incomes to the settlers, the social costs and the disillusion, suspicion, inactivity and the eventual migration of some people from the settlements.

The Volta resettlement operation has been described as a brave and imaginative attempt with limited resources to tackle a challenge and an urgent crisis. The factors which influenced decisions in the resettlement programme have been listed as a reasonable time span, adequate administrative capacity, political support, sufficient finance and an absence of prior commitment. It has been suggested that one of the chief lessons that could be learnt from the Volta resettlement experience is the importance of not just mobilizing and being aware of alternatives but of ensuring conditions, particularly enough time, for the choice to be made between them[17].

With regard to the Community Health Programmes in the settlements, health posts were established where sick people could come for treatment.

The environmental health problems were such that it was soon realized that it was not enough to deliver health care to the people receiving it; rather they should be activated and organized so as to be able to participate in the activities that are involved in their receiving health care. Thus through community development and self-help projects, some villagers are participating in the schistosomiasis control programme, by providing for themselves safe water supply and good sanitary facilities. As multi-purpose health workers, the paramedical personnel have proved very useful in implementing the health programmes. We are trying in our rural health programme to find out how to use this cadre of health workers effectively and efficiently. The role and function of the paramedical personnel in rural health care are also the subject of research in the Danfa comprehensive rural health project of the Department of Community Health at the Ghana Medical School in Accra[18].

The role and function of the doctor in community health care, particularly in the rural areas, need considering carefully, for the traditional training of the doctor does not seem to prepare him for rural community health care programmes where he would have to assume the role of a manager and leader of the Community Health Team and also of the resources of the community. The Ghana Medical School is now implementing an educational programme that would prepare the students for the role they will have to fill in such situations. What one would like to see in the future is the Medical School involved in educating the entire health team, thus fostering the spirit of teamwork which is a key to any effective rural health system.

Since the Medical School and the Health Ministry have a common concern in the delivery of health services, the integration of programmes and of all cadres of health personnel is important. One way of achieving this is by field educational programmes: that is, integration from below rather than from above. This approach, however, requires a special orientation, guidance and tact.

El Batawi: A good example of community participation is the WHO-assisted onchocerciasis programme in which every village community participates by organizing groups called 'onchocerciasis control committees', made up of local people; they work with paramedical personnel and with health assistants. This is the nucleus from which the programme starts. I agree that the Chinese experience of the barefoot doctor and the participation of the community is an excellent example.

The lesson learned from the Volta Project and the health problems associated with man-made lakes have helped a great deal when a similar problem was faced in the Sudan after the High Dam was built at Aswan, and the Nasser Lake was developed. Large numbers of people had to move. When people moved from their original houses they went to newly built villages where the housing projects were much better than in their original habitat. This experiment, although small, demonstrated that you can do something about resettling people, and improving their living conditions, on occasions of this kind.

Dickinson: I have visited some of the new settlements of the Volta River Project. The location of the villages is usually admirable from the planners' point of view but not necessarily so from the point of view of the inhabitants. People are having to grow unfamiliar crops in soil they are not used to and which they do not know how to protect. They have little or no access to existing markets, nor do they have access to the usual middlemen on whom Ghanaian villagers depend to organize marketing, and to help them with loans in times of difficulty. Much the same has happened to the fishermen: they have very nice villages but all too often have found no fish in adjacent reaches of the lake. So, naturally, they have moved to where they can catch fish and have erected shanty dwellings nearby. Moreover, they were mostly river fishermen, and their traditional techniques are not necessarily those required for lake fishing; again, they have had to look for areas more familiar to them. There are a number of general factors, purely to do with the technologies of survival, which are missing in most of the sample of Volta Scheme villages I have seen.

A second point concerns the idea of an integrated approach to social development, and the utilization of medical resources in China has been mentioned. In China, unlike in most other countries, being a barefoot doctor enables you, if you are keen, to become a nurse, a technician, or even a doctor, because the progression to a doctor is from somebody who is interested, into somebody who helps and becomes a nurse, who takes further courses in training, and one day is recognized as a doctor's assistant. I think I may say, safely, that medical education in China is slightly less parochial than the system is in Britain and that it may be better suited to the needs of poor developing countries.

Illich: Dr Derban said that there are two ways of integrating, from above and from below. A rather controversial programme was started in the University of Mexico two years ago by some young men. It prepares health professionals. The organizers knew that at any Latin American university at least 20% of people will drop out every year. To ensure the utilization of drop-outs, a new device was invented. If you drop out after the first year, you get a very high-sounding title. If you drop out after two years, you get a little less high-sounding title; if you drop out of the third year, you are just an 'ecological medical assistant', but you can do legitimately practically everything by which Mexican doctors can make money!

References

1. POPULATION CENSUS OF GHANA (1960, 1970) Central Bureau of Statistics, Ghana
2. BIRMINGHAM, W., NEWSTADT, I. & OMABOE, E. N. (1966-1967) *A Study of Contemporary Ghana* (vol. 1, *The Economy of Ghana;* vol. 2, *Some Aspects of Social Structure*), Allen & Unwin, London
3. DERBAN, L. K. A. (1968) *An Outbreak of Arsenic Poisoning in a Gold Mine (mimeographed)*, Ministry of Health, Accra
4. DERBAN, L. K. A. (1974) An outbreak of food poisoning due to alkylmercury fungicide. *Archives of Environmental Health 28*, 49-52
5. ACKERMAN, W. C. *et al.* (1973) *Man-made Lakes: their Problems and Environmental Effects* (Geophysical Monograph no. 17), American Geophysical Union, Washington D.C.
6. TAYLOR, B.W. (1973) People in a rapidly changing environment: the first six years at Volta Lake. In *Man-made Lakes: their Problems and Environmental Effects* (Geophysical Monograph no. 17), American Geophysical Union, Washington D.C.
7. *Volta Resettlement Symposium Papers* (1965) Volta River Authority, Accra
8. KALITSI, E. A. K. (1973) Volta Lake in relation to the human population and some issues

in economics and management. In *Man-made Lakes: their Problems and Environmental Effects* (Geophysical Monograph no. 17), American Geophysical Union, Washington D.C.

9. *Volta Lake Research Report* (1971) UN Development Programme, Food and Agriculture Organization, Rome

10. KUZOE, F. (1974) *Insect Vectors of Diseases in the Lake – an Entomological Report on the Volta Lake.* Volta Lake Research and Development Project, Volta River Authority, Accra

11. OBENG, L. E. (1973) Volta Lake: physical and biological aspects. In *Man-made Lakes: their Problems and Environmental Effects* (Geophysical Monograph no. 17), American Geophysical Union, Washington D.C.

12. MURRAY, R. & DRAKE, R. (1970) *Relocation of Government Work: Personal, Social and Behavioural Issues* (The Tavistock Institute of Human Relations, HRC 490)

13. MURRAY, H. *et al.* (1970) *The Location of Government Review: Human Aspects of Dispersal* (The Tavistock Institute of Human Relations, HRC 517)

14. MURRAY, H. & DE BERKER, P. (1973) *Some Human Aspects of Civil Service Dispersal* (The Tavistock Institute of Human Relations, HRC 824)

15. CURLE, A. & TRIST, E. L. (1947-1948) Transitional communities and social re-connection. *Human Relations 1*, nos. 1 and 2

16. FRANKENBERG, R. & LEESON, J. (1974) in *Sociology and Development* (de Kadt, E. & Williams, G., eds.), Tavistock Publications, London

17. CHAMBERS, R. (ed.) (1970) *The Volta Resettlement Experience*, Pall Mall Press, London

18. *The Danfa Comprehensive Rural Health and Family Planning Project*, Accra, Ghana. Proceedings of the Vth Annual Review Meeting (1970) School of Public Health, University of California, Los Angeles

Industrial growth and nutrition

M. BAVANDI

The process of development has often been treated as synonymous with the economic growth of which, almost invariably, industrial growth has been an indispensable component. For many years the concept of development has been studied (and in some countries is still being studied) in terms of mathematically neat models that, while focussing on investment in non-human resources and using the criterion of an increase in material wealth, have failed to consider investment in human resources. In other words, in these models expenditure on food, education and health is considered as consumption, and is often neglected in development programmes. Even when good nutrition is stated as an objective in such programmes, its relative priority is overlooked when funds and resources are being allocated.

One reason for this attitude has been the lack of hard data which show the impact of nutrition on the development process. Berg and Muscat[1], however, believe that economic planners have insisted much more on the exact measurement of the impact of nutrition when allocating funds than they do when allocating large sums in other fields.

However, the thinking of economic planners has changed to some extent recently. This change in attitude may be due, in part, to the fact that national output in developed countries, in relation to investment, has been large when compared with that in developing countries. This could be attributed to better knowledge and hence good health, adequate education and, of course, satisfactory nutrition[1,2].

As the positive effects of good nutrition on development have begun to be realized, the old concept that national development programmes will ultimately result in good health and better nutrition has been challenged also. While increased economic well-being is believed to pave the road to better health and good nutrition, it is accepted now that good nutrition contributes to, and is an essential component of, development programmes. In this respect the effects of nutrition and economic development are mutual. In other words, nutrition can be the cause, rather than being simply the result, of development. This would imply that development should not be measured in narrowly conventional terms such as Gross National Product (GNP), investment, and rate of transfer of potential wealth into material capital but rather in terms of an improvement and enrichment of the quality of life of ordinary people through better eating and a more prosperous style of living[3,4].

INTERRELATIONSHIP OF NUTRITION AND INDUSTRY IN DEVELOPMENT PROGRAMMES

The contribution of nutrition

In the past ten years many research workers have attempted to analyse the relationship between nutrition and national development. Much has been done to demonstrate the effect of nutrition on both physical and mental development, because manpower and its quality make up the main ingredient in development programmes. It is now well established that inadequate nutrition, especially in childhood, adversely affects physical and mental development— often causing irreversible damage—and results in reduced physical performance and mental ability[5]. The impact of inadequate nutrition in adulthood shows itself in the form of an increased rate of absenteeism from work, lethargy, lack of drive, and increased morbidity among the labour force. Industrialists seem now to be convinced that better feeding of their workers, either because of improved nutritional status or through better motivation, will increase productivity. They seem, Weisberg[6] concludes, to have realized better than economic planners the old precept that 'an army marches on its stomach'. This subject has been reviewed recently[6].

Other workers have demonstrated the direct and short-term effects of nutrients on working performance. For example, iron supplementation of the diet has been shown to increase the working capacity of workers several times, by correcting the prevailing iron-deficiency anaemia. Calculated quantitatively, the benefit-to-cost ratio of correcting the anaemia has been estimated to be 260:1 by Basta and Churchill[7]. The effect of glucose supplementation in reducing factory accidents is demonstrated in another study[8].

The impact of industry

Analysis of the situation in industrially advanced countries shows clearly the direct relationship between industrialization and the general social well-being of people. But one has to be very cautious in concluding anything from these analyses, because the situation that exists now in the developed world is the result of a long-established, slow and balanced process of development over many years. It was a very different process from the unbalanced development strategies that are in vogue in many developing countries today. In the latter group the emphasis is usually on the development of a rather sophisticated, capital-intensive industry as the shortest and most rapid way to compensate for backwardness and to reach the largest possible GNP. This means changing rather abruptly from a traditional agriculture to an industry-based economy and consequently investing considerable sums in moderate or large-scale industrial schemes. In many countries funds have to be provided by or drained from the agricultural sector. The immediate outcome will be a switch in agriculture policy from food production to cash crops, in order for the country to be able to obtain foreign exchange. In the later stages, when home industry expands and gains momentum, food production becomes even more depressed because of the increasing demand for crops to be used as raw materials for industry. In any case, agriculture in general and food production in particular lose their former priority. In this fascination with industrialization, while the cultivation of crops like cotton, tobacco and cocoa is encouraged and agriculture becomes oriented towards industry, the question which often remains unanswered—and may also be unasked—is: where is the *food* to come from?

The social impact of industrialization and its direct effects on the nutrition of people are similar to those of urbanization. Some of the major consequences related to nutritional status include changes in food habits and feeding practices, the deprivation of the young mother of the help and knowledge of family members, including ignorance of breast-feeding, and the lack of enough money with which to buy nutritious foods.

However, although the unbalanced growth and expansion of industry may have harmful effects on the production of food, the beneficial aspects should not be ignored. Most important here is the expansion of the food industry, because of its double impact on nutrition. First, the food industry can increase the availability of food, through modern techniques of preservation; it can contribute to the distribution of processed food seasonally as well as geographically, and can prevent large losses, either through preservation or through the conversion of inedible parts to edible ones; finally, it can introduce new foods. Second, expansion of the food industry increases the demand for agricultural products and can enhance the production of food crops, creating new dimensions of demand and new market opportunities. In the latter respect not only is the supply of food increased but income is generated among those involved in the various stages from farm to mouth.

Unfortunately, experience in developing countries has shown that the outcome has not generally been in accordance with these expectations, and industrially processed food products have failed to reach a significant number of the needy population. The prospect of the food industry in developing countries will remain the same unless some dramatic changes are made[9]. However, one aspect which has not suffered from the common commercial constraints is fortification technology, especially with respect to cereal staples, and when governments have devoted money and energy to it.

The trend in the past decade in the developing world has shown that the process of development in these countries, which is largely based on industrial growth, although very successful in making the rich richer, has failed to diffuse prosperity, and of course good nutrition, among those who need it most. Unless positive measures are taken to break the chain of events making up the vicious cycle of: poor nutrition—retarded growth—lower skilled performance—less productive workers—poor economic situation—poor nutrition, the benefits of industrial growth will by-pass this cycle without interfering with events and without breaking the chain. It is obvious that since in the conventional theory of economic development, as pointed out earlier, expenditure on nutrition, health and education is considered to be consumption, while expenditure on industry is considered as investment, and since consumption displaces investment, they inevitably compete for the funds in the process of development.

The situation in almost the entire developing world, with the exception of South Korea and Taiwan, has been the same[10]. In Brazil in the last ten years, in spite of an increase in GNP per head of 2.5%, the share of the poorest 40% of the population has declined from 10% to 8% of the GNP. In Mexico during the past twenty years the *average* income per head has grown at a rate of 3% per year. Of this the richest 10% of the population increased their share from 49% in 1959 to 51% in 1969, while the share of the poor 40% declined from 14% to 11% and that of the poorest 20% decreased from 6% to 4% in 1969. This state of development is unacceptable and is growing more so in most of the developing world today[11]. The case of the oil-producing countries is rather different from that of the others. Here the large revenues from oil could mask the shortcomings of other sectors.

The situation in Iran, however, does not lie at the extreme of this spectrum. The country has undergone a rapid course of development and industrialization. Fig. 1 illustrates the trend in the increase of Gross Domestic Product (GDP) during the decade ending in 1972. The components of the GDP are given in

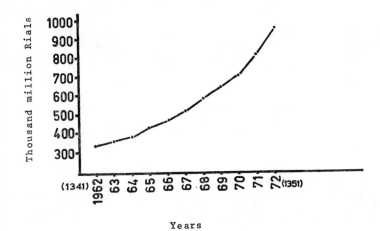

FIG. 1. Changes in Gross Domestic Product in Iran from 1962 to 1972. (Source: Fifth Development Plan of Iran, Plan & Budget Organization, Tehran.)

Table 1. It is apparent that while the increase in GDP seems quite satisfactory, the share of agriculture has dropped from 26.6% to 13.8% and has been replaced mainly by that of industry, which has increased from 17% to 21% of the GDP in 1972. Of particular interest and significance are the shares of the two sectors in terms of net figures and of rates of growth—the latter being 4% for agriculture and 14% for industry. Employment in agriculture and industry has followed the same pattern of change, decreasing from 55% to 40% in agriculture and increasing from 20% to 30% in industry.

TABLE 1

The components of the Gross Domestic Product in Iran (Source: Fifth Development Plan of Iran, Plan & Budget Organization, Tehran)

| Sector | GDP in 1962 | | GDP in 1972 | | % growth |
	Thousand million Rials	% of GDP	Thousand million Rials	% of GDP	
Agriculture	88.3	26.6	134.5	13.8	4
Industry	57.8	17	196	21	13.8
Services	117.5	35	372	38	15
Oil	67.3	20.3	271	27	15
	331		973.5		

TABLE 2

Distribution of employment in the main sectors of the economy in Iran in the period 1962–1972 (Source: Fifth Development Plan of Iran, Plan & Budget Organization, Tehran)

Sector	Numbers employed (thousands)		
	1962	1967	1972
Agriculture	3672 (55.1%)	3861 (49%)	3659 (40%)
Industry	1400 (20.7%)	1993 (25.3%)	2730 (30%)
Services	1584 (23.8%)	2020 (25.7%)	2740 (30%)

Table 2 illustrates changes in employment in the main sectors of the economy during the last ten years. In this period the population has increased from 23 millions in 1962 to 31.2 millions in 1972. The rate of increase of the urban population was 5.1% per year, which is considerably greater than the rate of increase of the rural population (1.9%). In absolute numbers the urban population has increased from 8 to 13.2 millions (from 35 to 42% of the total) in 1972. Most of the immigrants from the rural area to the urban areas have been employed as unskilled workers in industry or construction.

The patterns of consumption of the population, with regard to their family income and socioeconomic characteristics, have been discussed elsewhere[12]. Table 3 summarizes the amount spent by rural and urban dwellers on food in relation to their economic state and their total family expenditure. It also shows the distribution, by expenditure groups, of families in terms of the employment of the wage earner. Activities such as mining, construction, transport and power have been included under the heading of 'industry'. The monthly expenditure of the family on food has been translated into the available energy per head per day, with regard to family size for each expenditure group and at a given price (the real market price, and the same price for rural and urban areas) for the main food commodities. As Table 3 shows, for the same money that urban families spend on food they get less energy and nutrients than their rural counterparts. This is because rural people eat more bread, which is the main source of energy and protein in Iran, while urban people eat a more varied diet. The total protein intake ranges from 42 to 131 grammes per head per day in rural areas and from 40 to 112 grammes per head per day in urban areas. The amount of animal protein varies between 12 and 30% of the total protein intake in urban areas and between 10 and 16% of total protein in rural areas. In addition the urban population spend more on non-nutritious foods such as soft drinks, tea, coffee, and so on.

In a study made to determine the adequacy of the diet in relation to family income it was concluded that urban families spending less than 31.0 Rials per

TABLE 3

The distribution of energy intake, components of expenditure and types of employment in different groups in Iran in 1971 (Source: Publication no. 316 of the Statistics Center of Iran)

Expenditure groups (Rials/month)	Less than 2000		2000-2999		3000-3999		4000-4999		5000-7499		7500-9999		10 000-12 499		12 500-14 999		15 000-19 999		20 000-29 999	
Items	Rural	Urban	R	U	R	U	R	U	R	U	R	U	R	U	R	U	R	U	R	U
Available energy (kilocalories per head per day)	1550	1500	2000	1700	2150	1750	2400	1900	2700	2300	3200	2400	3750	2800	4100	2950	4315	3300	5700	3800
Expenditure on food (Rials per head per day)	10	11	15	13.5	16	14.5	18	17.5	20.5	20.5	25.5	24.5	29	28.5	32	30.5	37.5	34.5	45	42.5
Expenditure on non-nutritious food (Rials per head per day)	1	2	1	2.5	2	2.5	2.5	2.5	3	3	2.5	3	3	3.5	4	4.5	4	5.5	9.5	15
Expenditure on items other than food (Rials per head per day)	4.5	7.5	5.5	8	6.5	9.5	7.5	11.5	10	15.5	14	22.5	18.5	29.5	26	38	30	50	55	78.5
% of population employed in: Agriculture	62	8.5	74	17.5	77	15	76.5	15	76	9.5	79.5	6.5	77	6	80	4	65.5	2.5	81	4
Industry	12	31	13	36.5	12	60	10.5	38.5	9	34	7	32	5.5	27.5	4	25	6	18.5	2	18.5
Services	26	60.5	13	46	11	25	13	46.5	15	56	13.5	61.5	16.5	66.5	16	71	28.5	79	17	77.5

head per day (US$13.0 per month) on food could not satisfy their nutritional requirements[13]. This fact is confirmed in the present analysis in terms of the availability of energy. In urban areas the amount of food bought is adequate in groups spending 10000 Rials or more a month, and spending over 28.5 Rials a head per day on food and receiving 11.8 MJ (2800 kilocalories) of available energy. In rural areas this level of nutritional adequacy is achieved by groups spending 5000 Rials or more a month, who spend 20.0 Rials and obtain 11.4MJ (2700 kilocalories) of available energy per head per day. Energy and nutrients were calculated on the basis of a constant and actual price for different food commodities as purchased by rural and urban families, for which data were available, but allowances should be made because of the disparity in prices between rural and urban areas, also for the fact that most of the food eaten by rural families is produced domestically at much less than market price. Since the quantities of available food were calculated on the basis of the food bought and reported in terms of money, this will also create discrepancies that are not in favour of the rural communities.

The nutritional status of low-income urban groups in Iran has been studied by several people and found to be inadequate, as assessed by the lower birth weight and by infant malnutrition[14,15] and by the lower birth height[16]. The socioeconomic characteristics of these groups correspond to the expenditure groups of 3000–3999 Rials per month and below of urban families described in the present paper. Among urban people most of these families are wage-earners in industry, construction and related activities (60% are in the expenditure group 3000–3999 Rials).

The cumulative percentage distribution shows that the number of families with inadequate nutrition has decreased in rural areas from 91% in 1969 to 80% in 1971, while it has decreased in urban areas from 78% to 71% during the same period. The situation that emerges from these figures and could reflect the picture, with some differences, in many developing countries, emphasizes again that in spite of successes in the growth of industry and in development programmes, the nutrition—among other social aspects—of most people is still far from adequate. In these countries, as the demand for food grows, so does the necessity of importing increased amounts of food. This in turn increases prices, and governments then often have to subsidize prices as a welfare measure. It would be interesting to calculate the cost of importing food and of food subsidies and to see what the result would have been if these resources had been invested, at the appropriate time, in the domestic production of food. I believe that the justification of a common trend might then be questioned. Specific questions are: would it not be better to invest more in food production well in advance and before acquiring modern industries, and

TABLE 4

Allocations to various sectors in the Fourth and Fifth Development Plans in Iran (Source: Fifth Development Plan of Iran, Plan & Budget Organization, Tehran)

Sector	Fourth Plan (1962-1972) Thousand million Rials	Fifth Plan (1973-1978) Thousand million Rials
Agriculture	77.0	380.0
Industry	103.0	352.0
Education	134.0	550.0
Health and social welfare	65.0	315.0

before becoming short of food? Is the expansion of industry justified at the expense of a depression in agriculture and in food production? Does the expansion of industry realize the ultimate aims of development programmes and does it enable poor people to participate in the process of development?

Some development planners still adhere to the idea that unbalanced development programmes will ultimately lead to equilibrium and to balanced programmes in which each sector will have its legitimate share and in which the poor segments of society will be actively involved. This theory might prove to be true in the long run, but in fact reaching a balanced state in this way will mean that many people will suffer during the transition period and certainly those in need will suffer more. This would not be a negligible cost.

Having more than twenty years of experience in development and a rapid rate of industrialization, Iran has realized this fact and has adopted a policy that aims to grant prosperity to the mass of the population and self-sufficiency in food production. In this programme agriculture, education, health and nutrition have been given priority. Table 4 compares expenditure in various sectors in two planning periods and demonstrates the changing pattern of emphasis towards agriculture, education, health and nutrition.

In conclusion, it may prove to be essential for all developing nations, when adopting strategies for industrialization, to aim not only for the ultimate outcomes in terms of theoretical economics but also to aim to generate income and distribute it evenly among needy groups, to involve them in the process of development, and to analyse the middle-term impacts on the poorest groups with a more humanitarian insight than before.

Discussion

Dickinson: Dr Bavandi has drawn attention to the fact that in developing countries the relation between investment in agriculture and investment in industry is of crucial importance in social development, measured in terms of nutrition, and in the strategy necessary to break into the poverty cycle. If one looks at the more densely populated countries the relevance of the disposition of capital investment becomes even more apparent. With a postgraduate student I have been doing a study[17] on Bangladesh and, in particular, we have been looking at what can be done in the way of industrialization or urbanization or planning in a situation where there are plenty of people but there is almost no capital. The only real possibility, without outside aid, is to increase the productivity of the land. We are recommending that Bangladesh should aim to raise its land productivity in the first place; if this can be done without displacing people, who still have their occupations, they can feed better, they will have their own personal surpluses, and there will be something to tax in the process of accumulating capital. The next stage is to grow agricultural crops as sources of raw materials for local manufacturing and processing industries. It is only as a result of the development of oil-based industries that the growth of alternative agricultural inputs for industry, such as sugars, starches and fibres, has been neglected. It is only in this way that indigenous industries may be set up to use the real resources of the country, rather than importing an alien industry that only looks good because someone else has it already. I am encouraged by Dr Bavandi's formulation of what can be done in Iran. I am equally certain that the key to the development of the predominantly agrarian countries is the understanding of the significance of land productivity.

Ramalingaswami: I am very much interested in Dr Bavandi's ideas. One wonders, for example, what nutritional advantages have been conferred on disadvantaged groups in India by the Green Revolution. Although until two years ago agricultural production had gone up, the impression one gets is that the frequency with which you see malnutrition in the community, especially in the deprived segments of the population, has not changed. I have seen no evidence that it has improved the nutritional status of those people whose nutritional status is in real need of improvement. This raises the whole question of distributive justice, and where the enhanced returns from production are actually going. And if you look within the family, there is an unjust, un-physiological distribution. What are the forces that determine what kind of food goes to the head of the family, to the pregnant mother, to the child, and so on? Micro-level planning and change at the level of the home has lagged far behind the macro-level efforts towards more production.

The second comment is on the cycle you mentioned. This is a vicious circle of *developmental* defects: it is not merely a question of nutritional but also social deprivation and lack of social stimulation, and it is part of a multi-factorial poverty syndrome, that leads to disorders of development, mental and physical. To what extent one can influence this merely by introducing a nutritional component without changing educational patterns or without raising the immunological status of the group is an unanswered question.

Finally, on the question of what industrialization in general has done to the patterns of dietary intake of people and how it is reflected in their health, the main theme seems to be, with some exceptions, that people tend, with industrialization and economic growth, to resort to calorie-dense foods; the bulk of the food gets less because of processing, the fibre content of the diet is reduced, and more fat and sugar is ingested. This is a distinctive pattern. There is an idea that some of the diseases that have increased in incidence in developed societies may have done so partly at least as a result of this change in dietary pattern. It is not a deficiency of one item, but a change in the whole character and composition of the diet, which no longer puts the gastrointestinal tract to its proper use. Burkitt's hypothesis about the relatively high frequency of diverticulosis, colon cancer, and coronary heart disease that characterizes industrialized societies indicates a link with a shift in the composition and nature of the diet[18].

Bavandi: I quite agree that the production of more food is not going to be the ultimate answer to malnutrition in developing countries. About the impact of education of the public, a study[19] from Tamil Nadu in India recently showed that when people are feeding their children or their family they follow a 'silhouette function'; that is, they judge the needs in relation to the physical dimensions of the subject, not his or her requirements, so they are not giving the food to those members of families who need it most. They think that the men need more food and give it to them, rather than to, say, the growing children. Until we can change this belief by education or by some change in traditional practices, the mere *production* of food won't be the answer.

Holland: If we look at this problem from the point of view of nutrition in a developing rather than a developed country, we tend to believe that bigger is better—the more a child grows and the bigger he becomes, the better for him. But this is not necessarily so. One of the major public health problems in the UK and in the US is *over-*, not under-nutrition. In studies of school-children in Kent[20] about 10% of children between the ages of 9 and 13 years were classified as clinically obese. And to qualify for such a classification they really did have to be fat! We found no child with evidence of malnutrition in terms of being poorly nourished or having evidence of any vitamin deficiency.

Secondly, it is important to understand that intakes of individuals change over time; we may now be following outdated criteria of what is a satisfactory intake. Studies by Durnin and colleagues[21] in Glasgow school-children have shown that the food and energy expenditure has decreased over the last ten years, probably due to changes in social habit. Because we are leading a more sedentary life, we may not require as much food as we believe we do, from information based on studies done at a time when we led a much more active existence. In the UK we have changed the criteria for the provision of welfare food subsidies and the consumption of these foods is being monitored through the National Food Survey. An interesting finding is that since free welfare milk was stopped in 1972, the amount of milk drunk by families previously eligible for free milk has not changed. This suggests that such families have reduced their expenditure on other things to compensate for the change in welfare food policies.

One final important point is that there seems to be a critical age when nutrition must be adequate. In the UK it has long been noted that there are large differences in height and weight of children associated with differences in social class. Children from higher social class groups tend to be taller and heavier than those from lower social class groups[22]. However, in studies now being made, the rates of growth of children between 5 and 11 years are very similar in all social class groups. It would thus appear that social class, and therefore perhaps poverty, is more important in affecting the rate of physical growth below age 5 years (L. Irwig, personal communication). Other studies have also suggested that nutritional status is particularly important at certain stages of pregnancy and less important at others.

Porter: Dr Bavandi's paper is an extremely interesting one, coming as it does from a country with the fastest present rate of growth of GNP in the world. It is right, and most of us accept, that aggregate measures of welfare such as GNP are not satisfactory. But there is a danger that the reaction will go too far. The condition for breaking out of the vicious circle is an increased production of food, or the production of goods that can be exchanged for food. In other words, one improves welfare, up to a point at any rate, by increasing production and increasing the output of goods and services. In an affluent society there may be legitimate doubts about the relationship between increased income and increased welfare. The connection is much stronger in poor countries. It is true that in the process of development agriculture becomes *relatively* less important, but historically it is not correct that the process of economic development and industrialization in developing countries has been accompanied by an absolute decline in agriculture. It has not grown as fast as other things, but one wouldn't expect it to, because the difference between a person who is well-nourished and one who is undernourished is not great in terms of food intake. One would therefore expect the major determinant of demand for food to be the rate of population growth. In India the production of food grains has increased by about 3 % a year over a long period, just about keeping pace with the growth of population, and the so-called Green Revolution has not changed that figure much. But it has meant that whereas until a few years ago increasing food production came about largely by expanding the area under cultivation, there is now more intensive production from existing cultivated areas. The benefits of the 'Green Revolution' should not be underestimated, although there may be undesirable side-effects. Unfortunately, there has not been much change in nutritional status, because agricultural production has just about kept pace with the population; the amount of food available per head hasn't greatly altered. In our concern for equity and for the under-privileged, which is at the heart of the development process, we should not forget that these problems are only ameliorated when people are enabled to produce more of the goods and services they need; and this is difficult to achieve. There is a danger that people may say that industrialization is bad and imply that there is some other substitute which will enable countries to develop. I don't believe this.

White: I was interested by Dr Bavandi's evidence on the difference between the effects of industrialization on poor and richer people in Iran. But there is an over-simplification in the distinction being drawn between industry and agriculture. You said, Dr Bavandi, that industry creates employment and that that was one of the good things about industry. I don't think industry *does* always create employment: very often it takes it away, because it does with imported machinery what people were previously doing with very little capital. A few people make cars, and many people who used to provide forms of transport are put out of work. With a gramophone industry, people who provided music in the public square or other entertainment are deprived of work. This applies in a wide range of industries. So one has to look for the types of industry that will give employment. Industries are often set up in order to make at home what has previously been imported—'import sub-stitution'; but surely, rather than looking at the list of imports to find items it is feasible to make in one's own country, if one imports all the necessary equipment and makes an indistinguishable product, one should instead look at the list of imports to see what function each one performs? For instance, if they are cars, the function will be to transport certain categories of people, or certain types of goods, along certain routes, or to enhance the status of the owners, or all three. Then, one should see how those functions can be performed by something else that can be produced at home with the appropriate amount of capital per worker employed—that is, say, about £500 to provide a work place for a worker—a job—compared to the several thousand pounds involved in most Third World countries today. As for the status function, which is so often prominent in imports, it might be decided that this is one function that can be left unfulfilled; or thinking about how it could be fulfilled differently might lead one into a quite fundamental area of discussion of how governments can influence how social honour is accorded, how status rewards should be distributed, and of whether one cannot short-cut the expensive chain of motivating people to work because they want a lot of money, because they want to buy luxuries, because then people will admire them.

What I am saying about the need for employment is also related to Dr Bavandi's model of the vicious circle of nutrition or malnutrition. He is substituting his model for an economists' model in which the provision of greater economic opportunities, and therefore increasing GNP, leads to better nutrition. I think you have to combine the two models, because it's only with increasing economic opportunities—it's only when they have some job to do—that people whose nutrition is better can do anything productive. It is no use having healthy people if they can't keep up their wealth by having some kind of economic opportunity. Much of industry takes away economic opportunities rather than adding to them.

Bavandi: I was trying to stress that in the usual trend of economic growth and industrialization this vicious circle is overlooked, and development programmes by-pass this cycle in a which lot of poor people are simply circulating without any attempt being made to break it. In most developing countries, when industry is started, some employment opportunities are provided, but you are not increasing the total number of jobs; rather, you are displacing the labour force from agriculture to industry. It might sound, in the economic planners' way of thinking, as if people are getting more money and improved positions, socially and economically, but in fact they have to pay more for things they need and may suffer all the outcomes of urbanization.

On Professor Holland's point, physically bigger individuals may not be good, but one wants first to enable people to fulfill their capacity for physical development. In the developing countries the effect of malnutrition on mental capacity, in terms of measured I.Q. and the cell count of the brain, is more drastic than in developed countries[23,24]. If you exceed that capacity you will have overweight people, but this is another problem! I agree about the decreased energy requirement: the recent WHO/FAO recommendation[25] has lowered the requirement for calories. In my tables I was showing the purchased calories, not those consumed, so the figures are about 15 or 20% higher than what people really need. Our estimate of energy requirements in Iran is about 2400 kilocalories, and 15–20% over that comes to 2800 kilocalories.

El Batawi: The vicious cycle may not always apply in chronic situations of undernutrition in developing countries. An FAO study found that the average calorific intake in certain parts of Asia amounts to about 1400 kilocalories per person per 24 hours, which is a low level. In spite of that, people are working and producing. I agree that in certain situations the cycle operates; for example, during the Second World War when food was rationed in Germany, the annual tonnage of coal mined went down as a result of undernutrition in a population originally having a certain level of nutrition.

The second point that was raised is the transfer of workers to industry, which is claimed to reduce agricultural production. With the modern mechanization of agriculture, however, it has been observed that there is a chance of increased crops, particularly with the use of fertilizers. This is fundamental for combatting undernutrition which may result from overpopulation in the future. The food industry also plays a role in improving the quality of food and combatting the problems of *mal*nutrition. Some modern food industries produce a nutritionally balanced diet in terms of vitamins, protein and calories, and that helps in ameliorating malnutrition.

Jones: A major nutritional experiment was the introduction of food rationing during the Second World War in the UK. This influenced not only the quantity but the quality of food, and its distribution to certain vulnerable groups. If we use a sensitive indicator of the nutritional state of the UK, namely a comparison of nutrition of school-children in the early 1930's and in the late 1940's, this was a wholly successful experiment. Whether rationing can be introduced in other countries and in conditions other than war time I don't know, but it was one of the most successful large-scale nutritional experiments made so far.

References

1. BERG, A. & MUSCAT, R. (1972) Nutrition and development: the view of the planner. *American Journal of Clinical Nutrition 25*, 186-209
2. BERG, A. (1973) in *The Nutrition Factor: its Role in National Development*, pp. 2-30 and 40-49, Brookings Institution, Washington D.C.
3. MELLOR, J. W. (1973) in *Nutrition, National Development and Planning* (Berg, A., Scrimshaw, N.S. & Call, D.L., eds.), pp. 70-74, The MIT Press, Cambridge, Mass.
4. GOPALAN, C. (1973) Nutrition and national development. In *Proceedings of the Second Regional Seminar on Food and Nutrition*, UNICEF, Beirut
5. CORREA, H. (1974) The measured influence of nutrition on personal and social development. *League for International Food Education Newsletter*, March 1974, pp. 3-7
6. WEISBERG, S. M., REES, K. M. & McDONALD, P. (1972) *Nutrition and Productivity; their Relationship in Developing Countries*, League for International Food Education, Washington D.C.

7. BASTA, S. S. & CHURCHILL, A. (1974) Iron deficiency anemia and the productivity of adult males in Indonesia. Staff Working Paper no. 173, Research Division, Transport and Urban Projects Dept, International Bank for Reconstruction and Development, Washington D.C.

8. BROOK, J. D. & TOOGOOD, S. (1973) Factory accidents and carbohydrate supplements. *Proceedings of the Nutrition Society 23*, 94A-95A

9. BERG, A. (1972) Industry's struggle with world malnutrition. *Harvard Business Review*, January-February issue, pp. 130-141

10. CANTOR, S. M. & MEISS, A. N. (1974) An overview of the international food and nutrition situation. *Cereal Science Today 19*, pp. 92-95

11. MCNAMARA, R. S. (1972) Address to the United Nations Conference on Trade and Development, International Bank for Reconstruction and Development, Washington D.C.

12. BAVANDI, M. (1973) Food control in relation to socio-economic realities. In *Proceedings of Sub-Regional Seminar on Food Control*, pp. 29-34, UNICEF, Beirut

13. GHASSEMI, H. & MASSOUDI, M. (1971) Food budgeting for adequate nutrition in Tehran. *Journal of the American Dietetic Association 58*, 219-224

14. SADRE, M., BAVANDI, M. & SADIGHE, G. (1972) Nutritional status of a group of Iranian mothers and children in relation to their socio-economic backgrounds. In *Proceedings of the First Asian Congress of Nutrition* (Tulpule, P. G., Kamala, S. & Jaya Rao, eds.), pp. 835-839, National Institute of Nutrition, Hyderabad, India

15. HEDAYAT, Sh., KOOHESTANI, P. A., GHASSEMI, H. & KAMALI, P. (1971) Birth weight in relation to economic status and certain maternal factors based on an Iranian sample. *Tropical and Geographical Medicine 23*, 355-364

16. HEDAYAT, Sh., KOOHESTANI, P. A. & KAMALI, P. (1971) Influence of economic status and certain maternal factors on birth height. *Journal of Tropical Pediatrics 17*, 163-167

17. QUAZI, AKEF M. A. (1975) *Urbanization and Rural Development*, Town and Country Planning Summer School, Exeter 1974

18. BURKITT, D. P. (1973) Some diseases characteristic of modern Western civilisation; a possible common factor. *Clinical Radiology 24*, 271-280

19. THE TAMIL NADU NUTRITION STUDY (1973) vol. 1, Sidney M. Cantor Ass., Haverford, Pennsylvania 19041, USA

20. COOK, JUDITH, ALTMAN, D. G., MOORE, DIANA, M. C., TOPP, SONIA, G., HOLLAND, W. W. & ELLIOTT, A. (1973) A survey of the nutritional status of schoolchildren. Relation between nutrient intake and socio-economic factors. *British Journal of Preventive and Social Medicine 27*, 91-99

21. DURNIN, J. V. G. A., LONERGAN, M. E., GOOD, J. & EWAN, A. (1974) A cross-sectional nutritional and anthropometric study, with an interval of 7 years, on 611 young adolescent schoolchildren. *British Journal of Nutrition 32*, 169-179

22. TOPP, S. G., COOK, J., HOLLAND, W. W. & ELLIOTT, A. (1970) Influence of environmental factors on height and weight of schoolchildren. *British Journal of Preventive and Social Medicine 24*, 154-162

23. SCRIMSHAW, N. S. & GORDON, J. E. (eds.) (1968) *Malnutrition, Learning and Behavior*, The MIT Press, Cambridge, Mass.

24. WINICK, M. (1969) Malnutrition and brain development. *Journal of Pediatrics 74*, 667-669

25. WORLD HEALTH ORGANIZATION (1973) *WHO Technical Report Series* no. 522

Health and industrial growth: the current Indian scene

V. RAMALINGASWAMI

Developing countries carry a double burden: the existing burden of poor health conditions consequent upon underdevelopment, the hallmarks of which are poor environmental sanitation, malnutrition and rapid population growth; and the evolving burden of new health problems consequent upon the adoption of current patterns of economic development. Alleviation of the former involves the determined application of known knowledge and technology through political will and that of the latter requires the simultaneous establishment of health protective measures to deal with the problems anticipated from industrial technology. The transition period can be very difficult. A health policy related to environment-centred preventive activities is of immediate importance; the health implications of economic policies require simultaneous consideration. The provision of clean water and the sanitary collection, treatment and disposal of human wastes are the prime needs; waste discharges, air pollution and occupational health hazards are added off-shoots of industrial growth. The problem for developing countries is therefore one of how to meet the challenge of a high pace of development. Concern for socio-economic development need not be a choice between poverty and pollution. A balanced and integrated strategy is needed. A qualitative improvement of life as a whole is the goal rather than the pursuit of single-dimensional models which equate industrial growth with development.

THE CURRENT HEALTH SCENE IN INDIA

Planning is considered an essential instrument of progress in India and is closely linked with science. Side by side with economic growth there have been improvements in the indicators of health over the past two decades[1]. The crude death rate per thousand of population decreased from 27.4 in 1941–1950

89

to 22.8 in 1951–1960 and is estimated to be around 15.9 for 1970. Life expectancy at birth increased from 32.1 years in 1941–1950 to about 50 years in 1971. There have been similar changes in the other indicators of health. There has also been over the successive Five-Year Plans the development of a network of basic health services for defined units of the rural population as a part of total community development. The importance of family planning was recognized and as early as 1952 India adopted family planning as an official policy and as an integral part of socioeconomic development. Much progress has been made in the control of communicable diseases.

Despite these advances the current health scene is a cause for concern. It is characterized by a cluster of causes and a multiplicity of effects. India's population was estimated in 1971 to be 547.95 millions, of which 42.02% belonged to the 0–14 years age group. Infant and child mortality rates are still high, compensated by high birth rates. The disease pattern in infants and children reflects the synergistic reaction between malnutrition and infection aided by economic backwardness, poverty, illiteracy and traditional ways of life and by severely limited resources to set against large and unsolved problems. The proportional mortality rate in children below four years is as high as 40% compared with less than 7% in developed countries. Seventeen per cent of children suffer from severe-grade malnutrition and 55% suffer from mild to moderate grades. Maternal mortality is high; the frequency of anaemia is as high as 40% or more in women in the reproductive age group.

A rapidly increasing population, urbanization, inadequate sanitation, microbial pollution and lack of protected water supply are the features of the Indian environment. The problems of safe water supply and sewage disposal are even more severe for the rural population. Only about 10% of the villages have protected water supplies. Disposal of wastes lags behind the provision of water supplies. The impact on health is revealed by the high frequency of intestinal infections and infestations, including cholera, typhoid, the dysenteries, hepatitis, and helminth infections. There is an urgent need for the use of low-cost methods of treating water and sewage suited to the local conditions of the environment, the habits of the people and climatic factors. Community water supplies and sewage treatment constitute the greatest challenge to public health in India today. In addition to tackling these, we are developing a strategy resting upon the tripod of Nutrition, Immunization and Fertility Regulation, in which health care of the mother and the child is used as an entering wedge for its implementation.

INDUSTRIAL HEALTH

While basic sanitary facilities are being extended to the majority of the population, the country is industrializing itself on a rapid scale and is now in a position to manufacture sophisticated electronic and other equipment, including nuclear power reactors. A fairly large infrastructure in industry and science and technology has been built. The bulk of the working population in India is still engaged in agricultural operations—nearly 120 million persons. Three-quarters of a million people are employed in the mining and quarrying industry, and five million in the manufacturing industry[2]. Although studies on the dust hazards in Indian mining, quarrying, sand-blasting and other industries are limited, they do indicate that the problem requires deeper study, particularly in respect of pneumoconiosis and silicosis, the major occupational health problems of the mining industry. The assessment of air-borne dust in a number of coal mines has shown high dust concentrations in many places[3]. Dusts from the Kolar gold mines in South India are known for the milder reaction they cause in comparison to those in other parts of the world. The lung pictures are also different from those of typical silicosis. Silicosis has been reported from lead and zinc, manganese and iron ore mines. Appropriate standards and techniques for dust evaluation in the light of the working conditions prevailing in Indian mines and industries are now receiving attention. A number of national laws and regulations, such as the Factories Act, the Mines Act, the Tea Planters Act and the Dock Labourers Act, have been introduced from time to time to protect the interests of industrial workers. There is also an Employees State Insurance Corporation which takes care of the general health of industrial workers and their families. A number of institutions dealing with industrial and occupational health have been set up within the country. There is, however, a paucity of specialists in industrial medicine working within industrial establishments. Preventive industrial medicine has yet to catch up with the pace of industrial advances.

There is growing evidence of pollution of rivers by the direct discharge of industrial wastes in India. The warm climate and high water temperatures in India have an adverse effect on the oxygen economy of water. Industrial wastes vary widely in their composition; they include plant and animal wastes, acids, alkalis, organic and inorganic chemicals, synthetic detergents, fertilizers and pesticides. The arid and semi-arid areas pose another problem because of lack of dilution of the chemicals. In the past, dilution and natural purification were sufficient but the population density and the industrial expansion require that waste water should now be treated[4]. Population growth leads to the concentrated discharge of large quantities of wastes into rivers. As society becomes industrialized traditional domestic solid wastes are augmented by industrial and agricultural wastes.

Indian agriculture is shifting in its emphasis from high-yielding varieties of seeds and chemical fertilizers to crop protection and the Indian farmer is poised for an increased use of pesticides to protect his crops during the coming years[5]. As against an estimated consumption of some 30 000 tons of technical-grade pesticides in agriculture in the year 1971–1972, the public health programmes are reported to have used only about 5000–6000 tons. The average per hectare consumption of pesticides is only 160 grams in India, as against 1000–10 000 grams per hectare in countries like Germany, the USA and Japan. The amount of pesticides used has almost trebled in India during the last decade. The situation is particularly difficult because the farmer has begun with the most effective and therefore the most toxic and invariably the cheapest chemicals and would find it difficult to give them up in favour of safer but perhaps less effective and generally more expensive chemicals. During the last three years the area receiving pesticides with the help of aircraft has increased from 446 000 hectares to 1.09 million hectares. The health hazards arising out of the extensive agricultural and public health use of pesticides need serious consideration.

The withdrawal of DDT at this time from public health use could give rise to immense problems and expose large populations to endemic and epidemic malaria[6]. One thousand million people are now living in areas where malaria was once endemic, and which are now free. There was first a report that prolonged exposure to DDT led to an increased incidence of tumours, of various sites and in succeeding generations of laboratory animals. Experiments initiated by the International Agency for Research on Cancer failed to confirm that tumours occur at multiple sites or increase in incidence in succeeding generations. At the lowest level, namely two milligrams of DDT per kilogram of feed or 0.3 milligrams per kilogram of body weight, which is similar to the highest daily intake known to occur in man, one centre found a significant increase in liver tumours in male animals only, and the other centre found no increase in liver tumours. The first report on the tumorigenic activity of DDT appeared as long ago as 1947 and in 20 years no adverse effects have been observed in heavily exposed men[7]. In the present state of our knowledge, any risk to man is out-weighed by the benefits arising from a controlled use of DDT. Studies in Brazil and India comparing spray-men, exposed to DDT for long periods, and controls for 15 years or more revealed no clinical effects of this exposure despite very marked differences in blood levels of DDT (Table 1).

India is also facing the problem of air pollution created by urbanization and industrialization. In a recent study made by the Central Public Health En-

TABLE 1

The concentration of DDT in the serum or whole blood of spray-men, formulators and people without special exposure to DDT (*source*: WHO Report[7].)

Location	Exposed men		Controls	
	Number of blood analyses	Mean level of total DDT (mg/litre)	Number of blood analyses	Mean level of total DDT (mg/litre)
India				
Preliminary survey[a]	44	0.761	27	0.051
Main survey	100	1.272	98	0.170
USA (formulators)[b]	20	0.737	10	0.07

[a] Results on whole blood specimens. All other results are on serum specimens.
[b] Data from Laws *et al.*[8]

gineering Research Institute, Nagpur, it was found that the problem of air pollution exists in four major cities surveyed and that in some parts of these cities it is comparable to that in the most polluted cities in the world[9]. This is particularly true of the suspended particulate concentration and the carbon monoxide and sulphur dioxide levels (Tables 2 and 3). It was found that the concentration of carbon monoxide resulting from automobile exhaust at street level in Calcutta varied from as high as 33 parts per million to less than 10 parts per million in certain selected streets. The level of carbon monoxide recorded in Calcutta is comparable to that in New York, Chicago and London[11]. Another factor in the Indian environment is the smothering smoke from burning cow-dung, fire wood and raw coal. Raw coal is used as a domestic fuel and contributes much to air pollution.

TABLE 2

Concentrations of carbon monoxide in the atmosphere in some major cities

City	Maximum one hour values (p.p.m.)
London	58
Chicago	46
Los Angeles	43
Washington	41
New York	27
Calcutta	35

TABLE 3

Levels of pollutants in some Indian cities

Pollutant	Quantity	Ahmedabad	Calcutta	Delhi	Jaipur	Kanpur	Madras	Nagpur
Sulphur dioxide (p.p.m.)	average	0.004	0.015	0.022	0.002	0.030	0.011	0.004
	maximum	0.010	0.066	0.130	0.005	0.060	0.018	0.013
Nitrogen dioxide (p.p.m.)	average	0.005	0.017	0.008	0.008	0.004	0.014	0.013
	maximum	0.011	0.056	0.019	0.007	0.012	0.060	0.031
Hydrogen sulphide (p.p.m.)	average	–	–	0.0002	–	–	0.004	–
	maximum	–	–	0.001	–	–	0.016	–
Suspended particulates (mg/m^3)	average	0.342	0.350	0.631	0.439	0.591	0.060	0.302
	maximum	0.505	0.663	0.997	0.114	1.567	0.103	0.546
Dustfall rate (tons per mile^2/month)	average	196	25	106	85	114	–	29
	maximum	283	37	195	101	283	–	40

Details are not given (see source, below) on the significance and comparability of these results. Since they vary with the time and duration of observations, sampling techniques, type of equipment, and the position of the sensor (especially its height above ground), the numbers given should be taken as being approximate.

Source: data from Central Public Health Engineering Research Institute, Nagpur, based on a five-year study in each centre. Quoted in ref. 10.

NATIONAL COMMITTEE ON ENVIRONMENTAL PLANNING AND
COORDINATION

A National Committee on Environmental Planning and Coordination was established in February, 1972 in India with a specific mandate: to identify and investigate problems of preserving and improving the human environment in the country in the context of population growth and its distribution and of economic development; to advise the Government and public authorities on the environmental repercussions of their activities; to review existing legislation, regulations and administrative machinery for environmental management; to coordinate environmental policies with economic policies and measures; and to advise on the conservation of nature in all its aspects. The efforts being made in this connection in India include the introduction of the Prevention of Water Pollution Bill; preventive measures for the control of industrial pollution, stipulating that in the letter of intent the entrepreneur should satisfy Government or a designated agency of Government that the design of the project provides adequately for preventing pollution, in accordance with certain minimum standards laid down by such agencies; a comprehensive approach to water management; an Air Pollution Bill; and a Pesticide Act.

CHOICES AND BLENDS

Each country has to establish its own path of development, and its own permissible levels of exposure to potentially dangerous materials used in industry. The general health of the population, its nutritional status, the geo-climatic factors and the living conditions must be considered. Mere enactment of legislation is not enough: its effective implementation has to be ensured. Countries in the process of industrializing have the opportunity of controlling industrial environmental pollution from the beginning by preventive action. The health consequences of industrial development can be foreseen and in-plant control measures and effective pre-treatment should be ensured. A proper blend of health policies directed towards the vicious circle of communicable diseases, malnutrition and population overgrowth and of health policies arising out of economic activities has to be evolved.

For India, the provision of *basic minimum needs* to the entire population is the immediate goal of socioeconomic development. It follows that the industries developed should be those that are essential to serve those needs. The simple processing of naturally occurring materials to meet local human needs still has a significant place. Rural industries could still be important in economic development in view of their capacity to create employment *in situ* at low capital cost. The National Committee on Science and Technology, along with the Khadi and Village Industries in India, has made plans in 1974 to improve the technology in a number of rural industries, such as edible oils, bee-keeping, bio-gas, and the increased use of inedible oil seeds. Intensive application on a large scale of science and technology for integrated rural development is the aim of the plan.

Often it is not the technology itself but its improper use that is to blame. At a time when edible oils were expeller-expressed, they were free from any toxic effects. When the oil mills launched a programme of large-scale solvent extraction of edible oils, it was imperative that proper food-grade solvents should be used, and the procedures adopted should be such as to leave no solvent residues in the oil. In 1966, many indigenous solvent-extracted ground-nut oil samples showed a carcinogenic effect when tested in animals[12].

The urban problem in India is becoming acute[13]. There are now ten cities with more than a million people in India and eight more are expected to attain this size by 1985. The existing 'million-cities' are already heavily over-burdened, with a totally inadequate social infrastructure. The rural migrant comes directly to the metropolis and the result is the squatter settlements which spring up on their own initiative and are fast growing.

The choices and blends depend upon the chosen path of development. The ingredients are large-scale industry, small-scale industry, rural industry and the adaptation of existing village craft to the new requirements. The health of the men at work and of the community around should be a central concern to all patterns of industrial growth. The microbial pollution of the environment of underdevelopment is compounded by micro-chemical pollution of the process of development. A holistic ecological system based on man and his environment is what is needed. Cities, towns and rural areas should be tackled simultaneously in a national policy on the spatial distribution of population[13].

Discussion

White: When you say that India needs a 'national policy on the spatial distribution of population', you seem to be thinking as a planner sitting above all the millions of people in India, rather than asking what you can do to provide people with better alternatives, *if* they choose to adopt those alternatives. Urbanization is surely caused by people choosing to go to a place where they can get a better standard of living than they could in the countryside. From my studies in El Salvador[14,15] this seems to be the basic reason why people move, and even more people might be expected to move for this reason but don't do so because there are other reasons restraining most people, such as a family connection.

The move to the cities is a rational response of people to their economic situation and in the cities they adopt the most rational ways of living that they can, building their own houses in squatter settlements, finding something to do when they can't get jobs through formal organizations, selling things and services. The solution for them, surely, is to provide facilities that will enable them to solve the rest of their problems in the way they want to, not to try to send them back home or keep them at home, except by providing a better environment at home; but also to provide this in the city when they get there—to give them a plot of land on which they can have a house and maybe some domestic animals or a garden; to provide basic services or the possibility of building them for themselves, such as sewerage and water supply. In general one should not look at people from above but ask them what their needs are, and organize them in committees so that they can do these things for themselves and only *provide* what the city has to provide.

Ashby: From my own—admittedly superficial—observations in Ibo country in Eastern Nigeria, I came to the conclusion that a major reason for leaving the countryside and going to the city was to get away from the hierarchical system of the extended family. A person who is a junior member of the village remains like that; his place in the pecking order in the village hierarchy remains low for as long as 20 years or more, until he becomes senior enough to command respect. One reason—though of course not the only one—for emigration into the towns was to escape this strict hierarchical discipline. A possible cure, therefore, would be to loosen the hierarchical system. In India, does this play any part in the move to the city?

Ramalingaswami: The main reason for the move to cities in India is economic. Perhaps to some extent the social organization and the caste structure might be involved as well, but it is poverty, basically, and the hope in the city.

In reply to Dr White, to plan is to foresee and also to meet people's needs wherever they happen to be—in their villages, in intermediate-sized towns, or in cities. It is in fact the intermediate-sized towns that are deteriorating most in India because of lack of support. They could be strengthened and the kind of facilities you mention could be provided there to serve as an attraction and to relieve pressure on cities. This is not planning *against* the wishes of people, to the extent that one knows them.

Papanek: City and environmental planners in Finland have found a radical solution for these planning problems. Admittedly it comes as a high technology solution from a fully industrialized country. Nonetheless it tends to show how people can articulate their own needs with planners on their side. When it was found that too many people in Finland were moving into Helsinki, the city planners of Helsinki began building opera houses, theatres, concert halls, parks and shopping centres in Turku, Jyväskylä and other cities of Finland. One can see that this approach might not work in the US or most of Western Europe. However, it has made it possible at least in Finland for people to find satisfaction and goals in the countryside.

Bridger: I doubt if it is a question of whether one has *either* paternalistic planning, *or* full participation by people in what is going on. One must be realistic; there is a limit to the extent to which people can, at the level of their situation and their knowledge, take part in decisions that affect them. If you postulate that people will take part in *all* the intellectual intricacies to which they are not accustomed, you will inevitably demonstrate that people are *not* fit to take part in planning. The problem is, to what extent one can balance and optimize the level and the area and the functions within which people can participate in decisions affecting their own lives? It needs the understanding and empathy that go with the kind of planning that can optimize the degree to which people can be enabled to think through their own problems.

White: My point is that people should be given opportunities, so that they can decide, in the sense that they do what is in their interest as individuals. At the same time one should try to involve people in decision-making in their local area as much as possible; but the main point as regards the distribution of population would be to give people opportunities to work in their home areas. This is a matter of providing small-scale industries throughout the country. One should also allow people to move to the city. Rather than have a plan which says that so many people must stay in the rural areas and so many people must or must not go to the city, one should have a plan stating that people must be given the opportunity to live where they want to live by providing economic opportunities there.

Porter: There seems to be a dilemma in so far as small-scale rural industrialization seems to be highly desirable on economic and social grounds while at the same time the health hazards in small-scale industries are considerable. From that point of view, a system, however desirable in other respects, of large numbers of small workshops scattered over a country the size of India would not necessarily be more physically healthy than one having larger concentrations of people in larger industrial units. Large units are usually healthier because it is easier to 'police' them than small industrial units. What you are suggesting will not necessarily lead to improved health, although it may be desirable on other grounds.

Jones: Have we enough information to say that small-scale industry is necessarily hazardous? In the UK, if we say that a small-scale industry employs less than 250 people in a factory, and that means about 80% of our quarter of a million factories, these have a somewhat higher industrial accident rate, but not enormously so. They are often filthy places, but we must not confuse aesthetics with morbidity! On the other hand, they are often, in my experience, happier places; but, again, we shouldn't confuse contentment with health.

Ramalingaswami: I don't think one can generalize. We have surveyed recently the metal ware industry in Mordabad, a town with a population of 250 000 in the state of Uttar Pradesh in India. Of these, nearly 40 000 are engaged in the metal ware industry, principally brass, which is essentially of the nature of a cottage industry spread over most of the town, one family generally confining itself to one process. It is not uncommon to see persons belonging to three generations working in one room, their ages ranging from 6 to 60 years. The environmental sanitation and working conditions of heat and light are appalling and there is a high morbidity related to respiratory disease, accidents, foreign bodies in the eyes, heat exhaustion, and so on (G. Joseph & J. S. Gill, unpublished observations, 1973).

Jones: A larger scale industry does provide, as an essential part of being large, a better standard of indigenous medical care.

Ashby: Are you talking about the same thing? Dr Jones is talking about an industry of 100 or 50 people; Professor Ramalingaswami may be talking about *five* people working in a back room.

Ramalingaswami: I am talking of small numbers of people usually on a family basis, at the cottage level.

El Batawi: In recent years WHO has coordinated studies in several countries in different regions of environmental and health conditions in small industries (with less than 50 employees[16]). In general the conditions of health in small industries, particularly in the developing countries, deserve special attention. The small-scale employees often face a variety of health problems; they are largely uncovered by labour-protective acts and enforcement and most of them do not have in-plant health services available. They lack the economic resources to deal with hazardous conditions in workplaces. There are also other social problems, such as lack of education and inadequate housing. A higher rate of morbidity due to occupational illness and other diseases is found in small factories than in similar types of industries of a larger size, and also higher accident rates. On the other hand, the face-to-face relationship between employer or owner and workers in small industries provides a psychological motivation and strengthens the identification of the worker with the work enterprise. I have seen instances where the workers may suffer from certain minor illnesses, but would still go to work because they are keen about it. Furthermore, the workers have a better chance of seeing the output of the workplace. This is a psychosocial factor that plays an important part in productivity.

Challis: It is true that you can 'police' large industry better, or small industries grouped together into industrial trading estates, as is done in the UK and could, I believe, be translated in its philosophy to Third World countries. 'Policing' is a mixture of giving information, because not all managements are capable of understanding what they have to do, and enforcing regulations. I think grouping of industries does help protect people from themselves, because of the ease with which they can be reached by the 'policing' authority.

Secondly—and we have found this even in the UK, which is fairly far advanced—small industrial concerns increasingly reach out for new chemicals to help them. The dangers lie in the misapplication of these chemicals, which are easily obtained once you have started industrializing. It is trite to say that full instructions for safe use are given on every package; people either don't or won't read them. One has therefore to watch for the spread into the smaller workplace of new chemical substances, as opposed to metalliferous or natural substances. This again means that if you follow Dr White's idea and encourage small local industry you should, from the point of view of health, concentrate first on natural industry—things like wood-turning or, as in India, brass-working—and make certain that as you introduce a more sophisticated but local industry it is under the control of people who understand the technology.

As a more general point, it seems that a key theme in the conference has turned out to be the organization and administration of population health services in countries which are developing. The industrial factor appears only as a symptom of a disturbed condition in society which has brought the health question into prominence. Urbanization is another symptom, and in many ways a more common one. The problems of the Indian subcontinent seem to be more intelligently appreciated with reference to urbanization and the consequential social structures, than with reference to industry.

Gilson: Although I would not underestimate the extra opportunities for hazards in small industries, one should remember that occupational diseases are generally rather well-defined and relatively easy to detect and to measure, whereas the beneficial effects of working in small groups with their high morale cannot be measured so easily, but, on the WHO definition of health, the gains may be very considerable. Because it happens to be easy to measure some of the ill effects, one should not over-emphasize their importance.

Sakabe: It should be pointed out that small factories use mainly batch processing, whereas large factories use automated flow processes, or the conveyor-belt system of production. The difference has its effects not only on physical health but on mental well-being. People prefer batch processes, because the worker can start from the raw materials and go through to the end product, and see what he has produced. The strategy of producing goods should take human beings into account and should recognize the value of the small factory. It is not only a matter of hygiene: the productive method is also important to the worker.

White: I said earlier that I thought it necessary to distinguish between one kind of industry and another. I would now add that it is necessary to distinguish between one kind of *small* industry and another. The kind of small industry I was suggesting that an underdeveloped country should encourage in its rural areas and small towns was an industry at an intermediate level of capital intensity, but run by municipalities or government agencies rather than through the encouragement of artisans who run small workshops. One should of course at the same time encourage artisans to adopt electricity and improve their levels of productivity, but that by itself will not provide sufficient local opportunities for everyone; one has to do it directly through government because private entrepreneurs will not be attracted to that kind of production in sufficient numbers. One has to control large-scale industries rigidly, but it is also necessary to have government directly instituting medium-scale industry.

As an example, of the (limited) role of the workshop level, in El Salvador I talked to a shoemaker who employed five people in his workshop; he said that there were hundreds like him in the city. When they introduced the social security laws, which provide for health insurance and unemployment benefit for a limited minority, the social security payments that the small employers in the shoe industry had to make were so big that it meant the difference between being able to stay in business and succumbing completely to the large-scale shoe factory. So while one may deplore the insanitary conditions and lack of social security at workshop level, it does provide employment; when the small workshops had to close, the employees were thrown onto the other low-level activities in the city—street selling, low-paid services and so on. Their addition to the large numbers of people already involved in low-level activities must have depressed the average productivity of all those activities; the more people in a line selling outside the market, the fewer items each person can sell. So in general the introduction of the social security law impoverished more people; which is an example of regressive government measures which present themselves as a public utility.

Porter: I was not intending to make any judgments about the desirability of one kind of industry, large or small; but it is a matter of stark reality that a great deal more small-scale industrialization will be a necessary, if not sufficient, condition for improving prosperity in many developing countries, and this has implications for the way in which preventive and curative health services are to be organized. The point to focus on is that there is a difficult problem of how to adapt the systems of curative and preventive medicine to different forms of economic organization and to a changing environment.

Dickinson: The concept of intermediate, or appropriate, technology can be brought in here. The term 'intermediate technology' was introduced by Dr E. F. Schumacher, founder of the London-based Intermediate Technology Development Group and author of *Small is Beautiful*[17]. I prefer to use the term 'socially appropriate technology', which is more explicit and less likely to be misunderstood[18].

It is not possible to give a concise definition of a socially appropriate technology but for any practical situation it is possible to imagine a range of alternative technologies that could provide the desired process or product, utilizing a range of differing inputs of materials, skills and capital. The final choice would take into account social and economic factors as well as those purely technical. From the point of view of a developing country not over-endowed with material resources it is necessary that a socially appropriate technology should:

1. Use readily available local materials and sources of power.
2. Minimize the content of imported materials.
3. Ensure that the quality and quantity of production will meet the continuing needs of the local or export market.
4. Ensure that the product can reach its final market regularly and without deterioration.
5. Use existing or easily transferable manual, technical and professional skills and minimize costly, complicated and time-consuming retraining.
6. Offer continuing or expanding employment prospects.
7. Minimize the displacement of labour or in any other way adding to the pool of unemployed and underemployed.
8. Minimize social and cultural disruption, especially to non-beneficiaries of the introduced processing or manufacturing unit.
9. Minimize the demand for capital from local or national sources.
10. Minimize foreign exchange requirements.
11. Ensure that capital is used in a manner that is compatible with local, regional and national development plans.
12. Distribute the main economic benefits in such a way that further productive investment is encouraged.
13. Ensure that the primary producer of agricultural products receives an adequate share of the value added by local processing.

There are several ways in which alternative technologies may be sought so that they may be tested for appropriateness. The first is to modify existing practices so that production may be increased or diversified without excessive demands being placed on available resources or on the structure of local society. Innovation at this level is likely to include the modification of traditional tools or machines, the introduction of new materials or new processes for well-known materials, or increased access to markets and monetary circulation. The demand for new products from the towns or attempts to substitute indigenous products for imports may well be the most important factors in stimulating the processing of agricultural products in rural areas. This is the more usual way in which economic, and consequently social, change occurs at village level, but by its dependence on a number of barely understood factors the process tends to be haphazard and difficult to integrate into wider economic plans.

The second way is to revive and introduce an older well-tried technology from an earlier stage of development of a different society or economy. This approach is particularly attractive, because earlier experience with a technology could be expected to lead to success more readily than would an untried innovation. There is here a difficulty that may be insuperable: while the technology may have been effective in the past it is unlikely that any records exist of the way in which it was integrated into the society that made use of it.

The third way is to invent a new technology or change the scale of a modern technology to meet the needs of a particular production situation. This is the slowest way in which to produce innovations and it also is the most costly in its demand for skills, including many that are unlikely to be available in a poor country.

Workers in the field of socially appropriate technology see their role as being sources of information on a wide range of technologies, from agricultural processing to medicine. Choice of technology can only be made by the potential users in the light of their intimate knowledge of local social, economic and political conditions. As the application of socially appropriate technologies develops it is to be expected that autonomous agencies for the dissemination of such technologies will grow up within the developing countries themselves.

In Ghana I was involved in the setting up, in the University of Science and Technology, in Kumasi, of a unit called the Technology Consultancy Centre. The Centre is the principal agency through which the University plays a creative role in the economic development of the country. Technical advice and assistance is offered to major enterprises, small industries and village craftsmen as well as to the providers of essential services such as clean water supplies and improved housing. The University provides the staff for the Centre. Service fees are charged on a basis which is within the means of those who seek advice—they may be based on a cash payment, on a royalty payment on production, or on a share of increased profit. The establishment of the

Centre involved support from banks and charitable agencies and trusts, and staffing has been helped by secondments of engineers and technicians from a number of British educational institutions.

The Technology Consultancy Centre at Kumasi has already been involved in a number of production ventures, including the local manufacture of steel bolts, glue, pharmaceutical products, simple looms and scientific instruments for schools. In addition repairs have been undertaken on hospital air-conditioning systems, X-ray apparatus, and road-vehicle testing equipment.

Similar centres are likely to be introduced elsewhere and, through either ITDG or university connections, I have been involved in exchanges of views with interested government organizations in Tanzania and Guyana, and universities in Mauritius, Zambia, Nigeria and Colombia.

El Batawi: At a level between manual labour, which is so prevalent in most developing countries, and automation, many industrial processes can be carried out using intermediate technology. This meets certain social goals in developing countries, particularly the problems of employment and job opportunities. With the introduction of intermediate technologies production can be increased and at the same time the chances for employment are expanded, particularly in overpopulated countries. This has been done in many countries where governmental institutions give assistance to small industries to develop their technological know-how and enable them to compete with larger industrial establishments. There have been some successes realized with the system, as in Pakistan where the Small-Scale Industrial Corporation assists cooperative schemes among employers, in marketing, buying raw materials, selling their products and improving their technology. They have also adopted some health programmes in an organized manner.

There are also the social security schemes which played an important role in Colombia and Venezuela, for example, which often deal with small-scale factories and provide medical care for their workers. There are several other ways of solving the problem. I have found, however, a number of incidents. For example, in Indonesia, I saw food factories that have been imported from Australia, with no machine guards and with inadequate handling of food products, resulting possibly in microbial contamination of food during the canning process. Old machinery is often bought because it is cheaper. In Sri Lanka, a tank for fermenting animal feed in one factory broke down a short time after being imported and used because it was rusty and worn out. I have also seen textile mills where the looms are noisy and dusty, with old carding engines, and these were imported from industrial nations and sold to industrializing countries. I have also seen the hazardous use of chemicals, including carcinogens. Dr Gilson mentioned the fact that you cannot measure psychosocial health as easily as physical health. While this is true, there are parameters by which you can assess psychosocial health, like absenteeism, production rate and labour turnover. In 1975, WHO plans to convene a meeting on the organizational patterns for the delivery of health services to small industries. Several patterns can be followed. In Singapore small factories are grouped in geographical areas, in what is known as 'flatted' factories—apartment houses where each apartment is a factory. When many small industries are located in one area, health services are more feasible and can be provided at lower cost. In the Republic of Korea the government has assisted small-scale employers by establishing occupational health centres, covering all aspects of health not only of the workers but also of their families. These health centres are supplemented by funds from employers and are highly effective.

Professor Ramalingaswami mentioned the use of DDT. I want to add one thing which I learnt about in 1973 when there was a shortage of DDT, which resulted in the recurrence of malaria in some South-East Asian countries. One reason was the reduced use of DDT, because of lack of funds to buy it. There has been a debate about the effects of DDT on health and whether it is carcinogenic. So far there has been no significant sign of ill-health among people exposed to DDT, although we know that it is stored in the body, in the fat, in high concentrations. It is unfair from the humane point of view to see that while with a relatively small amount of money a good deal of suffering and ill-health can be prevented, at the same time some highly industrialized countries are spending billions of dollars every year on armaments. There are also major droughts in Africa, and Asia, as other examples of injustice in the distribution of available resources in the world. I wonder how and when humanity can reach a stage of maturity at which it will use the resources of technology and raw materials for the purposes of health and peaceful living?

References

1. RAMALINGASWAMI, P. & RAMALINGASWAMI, V. P. (1973) India. In *Health Service Prospects: an International Survey* (Douglas-Wilson, I. & McLachlan, G., eds.), pp. 185-209, *The Lancet* & The Nuffield Provincial Hospitals Trust, London
2. Pocket Book of Labour Statistics (1974) Labour Bureau, Ministry of Labour, Government of India, Simla
3. CHAKRABORTY, M. K. (1970) The Indian Association of Occupational Health. *Indian Journal of Industrial Medicine 16*, 41-59
4. WORLD HEALTH ORGANIZATION (1968) Water pollution control in developing countries. *Technical Report Series* no. 404
5. CENTRAL INSECTICIDES BOARD (1972) A note prepared by the Secretary of the Board, July 1972

6. WORLD HEALTH ORGANIZATION (1973) Safe use of pesticides. *Technical Report Series* no. 513

7. WORLD HEALTH ORGANIZATION (1973) Health hazards in the working environment. *WHO Chronicle 27*, 344-346

8. LAWS, E. R., CURLEY, A. & BIROS, B. (1967) Men with intensive occupational exposure to DDT. A clinical and chemical study. *Archives of Environmental Health 15*, 766-775

9. SETH, G. K. (1971) *Environmental Degradation.* Paper from the Central Public Health Engineering Research Institute, Nagpur

10. NATIONAL COMMITTEE ON POLLUTION (1972) Report

11. RAMACHANDRAN, K. V. (1973) Monitoring air quality in New Bombay and its environment. In *Proceedings of a Symposium on Environmental Pollution*, pp. 267-278, Central Public Health Engineering Research Institute, Nagpur

12. RANADIVE, K. J., GOTHOSKAR, S. V. & TEZABWALA, B. U. (1972) Carcinogenicity of contaminants in indigenous edible oils. *International Journal of Cancer 10*, 652-666

13. VERGHESE, B. G. (1974) The inadvertent city. *The Hindustan Times Weekly*, June 16, p. 4

14. WHITE, A. (1973) *El Salvador*, Ernest Benn, London & Tonbridge, and Praeger, New York & Washington D.C.

15. WHITE, A. (1969) The social structure of the lower classes in San Salvador, Central America. PhD Dissertation, University of Cambridge

16. EL BATAWI, M. A. (1974) The forgotten masses. *World Health*, July-August 1974, pp. 4-9

17. SCHUMACHER, E. F. (1973) *Small is Beautiful*, Blond & Briggs, London

18. DICKINSON, H. (1972) *Dissemination of Appropriate Technologies*, Deutsche Stiftung für Entwicklungslander, International Workshop, Kumasi, Ghana

The impact of industrial growth on health in South-East Asia

W. O. PHOON

By 'South-East Asia' is usually meant the area consisting of the East Indies and the Indochinese peninsula of continental Asia. The term is usually taken to include the countries of Indonesia, Philippines, Singapore, Malaysia, Brunei, Burma, Thailand, Cambodia, Laos and Vietnam. The area contains approximately 250 million people. From the 16th to the first half of the 20th century all the constituent parts of the region were colonies of western powers, with the single exception of Thailand. By 1963, however, all parts of South-East Asia had gained their independence except Portuguese Timor. Brunei remains a British Protectorate.

The climate is predominantly tropical, with an annual rainfall generally above 40 inches (1000 mm). Rice and maize are the main staple foods. The region is very rich in natural resources, and produces rubber, rice, sugar, teak, tin, pepper, bauxite, petroleum, palm oil and coconut oil.

Industrial development in the region, as a whole, is still at an early stage. However, it varies greatly, ranging from Singapore, which is quite highly industrialized, with over 4000 factories, to Laos, which has virtually no major industry.

No matter at what stage of industrial development, all the governments in the region subscribe to a belief that industrialization is a prerequisite for progress and prosperity. This has been aptly expressed by Myrdal, although in the context of South Asia and not South-East Asia:

'It is reasonable that a discussion of economic development policies in South Asia should begin with the ideology of industrialization. A clamor for industrialization is notable in all countries of the region: when the intellectually elite say their countries are underdeveloped, they mean, in the first instance, that they have too little industry. Thus spokesmen for the South Asian

107

Countries frequently use the terms 'pre-industrial' or 'under-industrialized' as synonyms for 'poor' or 'undeveloped'"[1].

The commencement, or the intensification, of industrialization is commonly mentioned in national development plans. The Second Five-Year Plan of the Federation of Malaya (now Malaysia) is a case in point:

'For the future, the importance of manufacturing to the Federation's long-run development and economic diversification can hardly be over-emphasized'.[2]

The declared purpose of industrialization is usually the creation of more financial resources in order to improve the standards of living for the people. More jobs would be available. More money could be spent on community facilities such as schools, health clinics, and hospitals. However, economic reasons sometimes take second place to emotional or political ones:

'Whether or not there are sound economic reasons for the establishment of secondary industries in a primary producer country, the will and desire to establish such industries usually increases as the country progresses educationally and in political stature. The fact that home produced raw materials are exported, often thousands of miles, only to be reimported in a manufactured, or processed, and more expensive, form is sufficient in itself to impel attempts to set up similar manufacturing industries within the basic producer country'.[3]

Most of the political leaders in South-East Asia and the social and other scientists who advise them fully realize that development does not consist merely of industrial growth. Rather, 'development may be seen as a process of improving the capability of a nation's institutions and value system to meet increasing and different demands, whether they are social, political, or economic'.[4]

They are also aware that industrialization and the concomitant process of urbanization may result in undesirable by-products as well as the desired products of more affluence and social amenities:

'With rapid industrialization, urbanization and physical redevelopment, new dimensions in health policy have to do with the Government's concern for a more integrated approach towards the improvement of the total ecological environment and therefore include attention and new legislation with respect to industrial health, water and air pollution, and other measures to promote mass participation in raising public health standards'.[5]

THE COST IN HUMAN SUFFERING

A common problem is to decide what is the acceptable price, in terms of human suffering, that should be paid for development. Another problem is the difficulty of visualizing things that have not yet happened and of persuading the decision-making bodies to divert funds from the primary purpose of economic expansion to measures against the pollution, adverse social repercussions and ill-health which may result.

The social scientist may be a voice in the wilderness when he argues that individual human beings are more precious than money or machines. The industrialist does not own his workers, but he does own his machines. In relatively socially backward societies, such as many of the South-East Asian countries, there is usually an over-supply of unskilled labour. The proprietor or manager usually gets off quite lightly financially if workers in his factory are killed or injured. Therefore the message, to be effective, has often to be directed towards their pecuniary interests rather than towards their social conscience:

'It is agreed that the primary objective of industry is to make money, not to do charity. However, let it be remembered that men are the most important resources of any factory. Any industrialist would be considered a fool if he does not keep his machines properly lubricated or regularly maintained, but only send them for repairs whenever they break down. Yet some industrialists permit managers, supervisors and workmen to suffer from ill-health ... which must have telling, adverse economic effects in terms of wrong decisions, poor morale and lowered productivity'.[6]

On the other hand, the community as a whole may be more affected by stories of human pathos than by the cold sets of facts and figures usually presented by experts in occupational medicine and safety. Who will not be moved by the following true story, which describes a common yet very tragic occurrence?

'I once was in a factory and I met a little girl with three fingers cut off. This happened from an accident from a circulating saw. Then I thought of her plight and I looked at the whole condition from the beginning. This girl was warded in hospital for about three weeks, was treated by doctors, was given medicine, then was given sickness absence, of course, during the whole period of time, and at the end she was given compensation and then I asked the manager of the plant, "How much does it cost to have a guard on this circulating saw?" ... I found it was one-hundredth of the cost of the disabilities that had happened to this poor girl'.[7]

Unfortunately, we are not told who paid the hospital fees—probably the state, not the employer. Nor are we told who paid the compensation—probably the insurance company, not the employer directly. The employer perhaps paid only the usual insurance premium, regardless of whether the injury had occurred or not. So he probably still saved money (his own) by not installing a guard!

Sometimes occupational accidents and diseases are caused by the lack of technical education or orientation on the part of the workers pouring into the thousands of factories newly set up in recent years:

'The rural education of the migrating youth frequently does not provide him with the skill needed in urban areas. Although technical education is more easily available in cities, the frequent preference for white collar jobs has resulted in only rudimentary provision of vocational and technical education, even in cities. Consequently, the urban youth is also ill-prepared for industrial employment ... Even when the migrating youth is not exploited in factory employment, he has to adjust to the fact of work dictated by the unfamiliar machine. He is often puzzled by the piece-meal nature of his work and disturbed by the impersonality of industrial employment'.[8]

As so many new factories spring up, there is a great shortage of skilled managers and supervisors who can provide proper training and supervision for the raw recruits. This, in turn, leads to more mishaps in industry.

No apology is needed for concentrating attention on the worker, as he is the one exposed to the greatest concentrations of harmful substances produced by industries as well as to the physical hazards of his working environment. A recent seminar in South-East Asia stresses this:

'The majority of developing countries are today determined to start with industrialization and to upgrade their overall economy as rapidly as possible with a view to securing a higher standard of living. A rapid industrialization however, produces far-reaching changes in society and affects practically all of its strata. A number of developing countries are now passing through such a transition period and are having to adjust themselves to the requirements of modern society ...

'Radical changes in the way of living ... a completely changed type of housing and social environment, and new working methods often lead to a deterioration of mental and physical health. The health problems resulting from the introduction of new industrial processes, and from urbanisation and mechanization, are complex, in this context. Of particular importance, because of its contribution to the economic progress of any nation, is the health of the worker who is exposed not only to environmental and other community health hazards but also to a variety of physical and chemical hazards in his work environment'.[9]

THE EFFECTS OF INDUSTRIALIZATION ON THE COMMUNITY

I shall not discuss the ill-effects of industrialization on the general community in detail. In South-East Asia, as perhaps in the rest of the world, it is extremely difficult to separate the factors of urbanization, and the radical changes affecting traditional religions, culture and customs, from the factor of industrialization in the causation of the dramatic transformation of most parts of the region during recent years. It is also perhaps true to say that we cannot fully quantify all the effects directly resulting from urbanization. As was stated in a book on this subject:

'In the large cities ... it is not the quantitative aspects of public health problems that are predominant. The macro-hazards of epidemics have given place to a complex of such micro-hazards as air and water pollution and other unsolved issues of sanitation. These, however, are not the only factors of urbanization induced damages to health. Others, as for instance, urban noise, the increased risk of exposure to carcinogenic substances, or the stressors of city life are all noxious effects endangering the health of town dwellers. In comparison with the mass destruction caused by epidemics, the micro-hazards seem to be of minor importance; still, they are by far not negligible if their chronic, often accumulative, effect is considered'.[10]

The inevitable migration from the country to the urban areas has led to the equally inevitable problems of overcrowding and the development of shanty towns, with their poor sanitation, abject poverty and malnutrition. Some of the capital cities of South-East Asia have shanty towns accommodating a quarter or more of their populations:

'The expanding industrialisation in traditional urban centres has further exerted a special 'pull' towards movement of people to cities ... the result has been industrial expansion in already overcrowded urban centres and the further migration of potential labour from rural to urban areas in numbers surpassing employment opportunities, thus creating two serious problems of overcrowding and unemployment'.[11]

The problem of migration from rural areas into towns and cities is universally recognized, but effective solutions are not forthcoming. Many have been proposed:

'How do we solve this problem? Can we say let us stop industrialisation and let us go back to the villages? We must industrialize and do it rapidly. The only solution, as I see it, is to industrialize the villages instead of the cities. Take the industries into the villages rather than having the whole of village after village migrate into industrial complexes in the cities'.[12]

In Malaysia an attempt is being made to stem the tide of rural–urban migration by paying more attention to the development of agriculture, so that both jobs and productivity could be increased. Moreover, agricultural development is viewed as a necessary adjunct to industrial growth:

'In a very fundamental sense agricultural progress is a requirement for industrial growth ... Planners still have much to learn about agriculture's role in economic development. But they are now in general agreement on the need to give high priority to both agriculture and industrial development in national plans'.[13]

THE DIFFICULTIES OF EXTRAPOLATION FROM EXPERIENCES OF OTHER REGIONS

We cannot merely extrapolate the experiences of community medicine or occupational health gained in the developed countries of the West to another area of the world such as South-East Asia. The climatic conditions, in the first instance, are very different. This is sometimes not sufficiently realized by experts either living in the region or visiting it:

'The basic hygienic evaluation of the impact of air-borne concentrations of chemicals in industrial atmospheres refers to temperate climatic conditions. Gross deviations of physical pressure, ultraviolet and ionizing radiation in the atmosphere of work sites may result in adverse effects from these chemicals even if their concentration is permissible according to the list of Threshold Limit Values ...

'Human volunteers exposed to 2% parathion dust at different ambient temperatures have shown an increased absorption of para-nitro-phenol, following their exposure to 28°–46°C'.[14]

Not only is the physical environment in South-East Asia different from that in the West, but there are also inherent differences in the population which may produce dissimilar reactions to toxic substances or physical stresses. For instance, many people in South-East Asia are born with deficiency of an enzyme, glucose-6-phosphate dehydrogenase. Since the first clinical case of this enzyme deficiency in Singapore was described in 1959[15] it has been found to be the commonest cause of kernicterus (severe jaundice with injury to the brain in newborn children) in Singapore and to be quite a common cause of haemolytic anaemia, precipitated by chemicals and other substances.

OCCUPATIONAL HEALTH PROBLEMS IN SOUTH-EAST ASIA

I shall now describe some of the occupational health problems that exist in South-East Asian countries. It must be stressed that knowledge about these problems is very scanty because of inadequate machinery for the collection, processing and analysis of data in most parts of the region.

South Vietnam

By 1971, industry in Vietnam had been developing for twenty years. There were 22 550 industrial enterprises which employed approximately 240 000 workers. Industries included agriculture, forestry, mining, construction and public utilities.

There are elaborate occupational health laws, including the provision for the obligatory employment of a nurse for industries employing less than 100 workers, and provision for nurses and part-time physicians for industries employing more than 100 workers; and also yearly medical examinations for all workers[16]. Unfortunately, however, these provisions are not usually observed. This sad state of affairs is by no means unique to South Vietnam. Some politicians seem to tend to 'solve' the problems of industrialization by merely wishing them away—by passing elaborate sets of legislation without providing for adequate enforcement.

Thailand

There were 320 cases of pesticide poisoning in Rajburi Province in the five years from 1966 to 1970, including 24 fatalities. In 1971 the province contained a population of 3789, comprising actual users and exposed persons, and was largely agricultural[17].

Thirty cases of lead poisoning were described in small factories, making or handling lead print-type or smelting and refining lead.

In 1969 lead poisoning occurred in children from families who manufactured sugar from coconuts, in the process of which they used the cases of worn-out storage batteries as fuel[18].

In 1965, manganese poisoning in a dry-cell battery plant was reported. There were 44 cases of varying grades of paralysis in employees working in the mixing and filling operation of the factory[19].

Indonesia

A survey among miners showed that one in 200 (0.5 %) had silicosis. Among carders in the textile industry, an investigation of 20 people revealed two cases of bronchospasm associated with their job, one case of repeated bronchitis and two cases of chronic bronchitis. Occupational deaths from pesticide poisoning have also occurred. The nutritional status of workers was found to be often unfavourable. 'The prevalence rates of such diseases, however, appear to be relatively low due to the lack of reports, insufficient orientation of the physician to make the diagnosis, a high labour turnover ...'[20]

'The most prevalent occupational diseases are pneumoconiosis and dermatoses. Occupational metal diseases, and some other industrial poisonings, have been observed'.[21]

The Philippines

Silicosis, lead poisoning, and intoxication from pesticides have been described. Cases of byssinosis have also occurred (personal communication to the author).

Burma

Apart from industries related to agriculture, the most important industries in Burma are probably those related to oil refining and the weaving of cotton and silk fabrics. We do not possess information on occupational diseases in this country.

Laos

There are small industries manufacturing cigarettes, matches, soft drinks and rubber sandals, and also sawmills[22]. We have no information on occupational diseases in Laos.

Cambodia

Some agricultural and village industries exist. We do not possess information on occupational diseases in Cambodia.

Malaysia

In a population of nine million in the peninsular part of Malaysia, there is a total work force of about 3.2 million. Almost 50% of workers are engaged in agriculture, more than 9 % in manufacturing industries, 3.5 % in the construction industry, 3.7 % in transport, storage and communication, and 2.2 % in mining. Although there is a wide range of legislation, certain sections of the working population are still unprotected. Problems of enforcement exist[23].

Cases of poisoning from pesticides, lead poisoning, industrial accidents in the construction and other industries, and occupational dermatitis in the rubber and chemical industries, have been described (personal communication to the author).

A SINGAPORE CASE STUDY

Singapore will be discussed in greater depth, partly because I am more familiar with its problems and partly because it is the most advanced industrially of all the countries in South-East Asia. At first sight Singapore does not seem to have many things in common with other countries in the region. Its land area is by far the smallest (584.3 square kilometres, or 225.6 square miles). Its population is only approximately 2 200 000, people of Chinese origin accounting for 76%. In fact, many of the industrialized areas in the other South-East Asian courtries share the problems of Singapore. Moreover, at the rapid tempo of development prevailing in the region, what exists in Singapore today will probably exist in the neighbouring countries within a decade.

There is no doubt that industrialization has conferred immense material benefits on the people of Singapore. Partly because of industrialization, the average income per head in Singapore is over US$1300 per annum, the second highest in Asia. The contribution to the national economy by industry is also rapidly increasing.

'Over the last decade, the manufacturing sector has grown considerably, whether measured in terms of output, value added or employment ... The manufacturing sector's contribution to GDP at factor cost has risen from 9 per cent in 1960 to 17 per cent in 1969'.[24]

It is interesting to recall that when the programme of rapid industrialization began about fourteen years ago, 'The unemployment problem appears to have overshadowed all other problems in Singapore and has become almost the exclusive reason for industrialization'.[25] The number of jobs created by industrialization has meant that unemployment is no longer the only or even the most important problem as there is almost full employment and there are approximately 60 000 immigrant workers in Singapore now, mostly from Malaysia.

Very successful public housing programmes and the provision of better

TABLE 1

Industrial accidents in Singapore

Year	No. of accidents reported	No. of fatal accidents	No. permanently disabled
1968	8147	109	703
1969	8714	132	731
1970	9682	159	886
1971	10 197	147	1072
1972	10 675	186	1474

community health facilities in the form of more doctors, nurses, clinics, and hospitals have been made possible from the fruits of the industrialization programme and have made Singapore one of the cleanest and healthiest countries in Asia.

However, Singapore has not escaped the penalties of industrialization.

There are over 4000 factories, employing an estimated total of 130 000 workers. The most urgent health problem faced by factories is the increasing number of industrial accidents leading to deaths and injuries, as shown by Table 1. This increase is out of proportion to the increase in numbers of workers and factories over the same period.

TABLE 2

Industrial accidents reported in Singapore in 1972 in different industries

Industry	No. of accidents (including fatalities)	No. of factories with more than 40 accidents
Building and repairing of ships, tankers and other ocean-going vessels	645 (8)	13
Manufacture of plywood and veneers	319 (2)	8
General building construction	295 (22)	544
Civil engineering construction	117 (3)	91
Stone quarrying	103 (2)	35
General engineering works	73 (1)	276
Manufacture and repair of industrial and agricultural machinery (including engines and turbines)	68 (1)	78
Spinning, weaving, printing and finishing of yarns and fabrics	66	14
Iron and steel rolling mills	62 (1)	2
Building and repairing of barges, lighters and boats	53	18

Table 2 shows the number of accidents reported for 1972 by industry and the number of factories where the total number of accidents exceeded 40. Figures in brackets indicate fatalities.

Occupational diseases have also occurred in Singapore. It is not possible to give an exhaustive account here, but some examples may illustrate the problem. There are some 23 granite quarries employing about 1500 workers in Singapore. In a 1965 survey, out of 1188 workers X-rayed, 8% had definite silicosis and 24% had suspected silicosis. A similar survey, concluded in 1971, found that 15% had definite silicosis and 17% suspected silicosis, out of 1230 workers X-rayed. The other industries in which there is exposure to silica dust are rubber powder factories, iron foundries, pottery works, sand-blasting operations and tombstone-making[26].

Interesting cases dealt with by the Industrial Health Unit in 1972 included an outbreak of dermatitis in an electronics factory due to a liquid soap which predisposed to photo-sensitivity, and an outbreak of hysterical attacks among female workers in a plastic toy factory. This was the first 'epidemic' of hysteria ever reported in factory workers in Singapore[27].

Other occupational health problems in Singapore which have been reported include lead poisoning, occupational dermatitis, decompression illness, leptospirosis, heat stress and psychological problems due to maladjustment to jobs[28], and rockfish stings in fishermen[29].

In a survey of 83 small factories, it was found that only 12 had satisfactory standards of sanitation and safety. These small factories have very scanty financial resources, a high turnover of labour, and often very limited management and training skill—all factors which predispose to high rates of accidents[30].

The widespread practice by large firms of contracting out dirty or dangerous work is also making the enforcement of health and safety legislation more difficult. Employers sometimes inform factory inspectors that the hazards of lead poisoning or silicosis 'no longer exist' in their factories because they have handed over the processes involving such hazards to contractors! The situation described below exists in Singapore as it does in Japan:

'One of the major problems of industrial health in today's Japan is the hygiene problems of the 'inner contract workers' who, though working within a certain enterprise, have no direct employment contracts with the enterprise itself ... It has long been pointed out that the manufacturing processes for which the inner subcontract workers are responsible are often dangerous and unhealthy ones with a high incidence rate of labour accidents and occupational hazards'.[31]

In 1969, I listed some of the factors which impede the progress of occupational health in a developing country. The factors were:

1. Economic development usually gets most of the money available. Occupational health measures do not usually receive sufficient government funds, as it is argued that they can wait until the industries are fully launched.
2. The lack of sophistication by workers sometimes leads them to demand more money to carry out dangerous jobs or increased compensation for permanent disability, rather than to demand that their working environment should be made safe.
3. Employers and workers may agree about the desirability of using safety equipment, but disagree as to who should provide it.
4. The characteristically hot and humid climate makes the regular use of personal protective equipment very uncomfortable.
5. The polyglot nature of many developing countries sometimes leads to problems of communication between supervisors and workers, and these in turn may predispose to accidents.
6. The lack of uniformity in health and safety standards in industries established by multinational companies in the developed countries sometimes leads to confusion in the provision of health and safety measures.

In my own opinion, these factors have contributed to the incidence of accidents and diseases in the industries in Singapore[32].

The ill-effects of industrialization on the general community are more difficult to determine. During the last few years there has been more congestion of traffic, more overcrowding, more pollution and an increase in the tempo of living. During the construction of factories, there have been occasions when mosquito breeding has increased because pools of stagnant water have formed. In 1973 there were over 1000 cases of dengue haemorrhagic fever in Singapore, some of which could be attributed to an increase in the population of *Aedes aegypti* mosquitoes on the construction sites. Psychiatrists have claimed that there is more mental ill-health in the community. In the report of a Committee on Crime and Delinquency, set up by the Singapore Government, it was stated that 'crime among the young had increased at an alarming rate over a five-year period from 1968 ... the crimes by juveniles against property with violence rose from 30 in 1968 to 119 in 1972'.[33] Suicide does not seem to have increased, though the mode of suicide has changed: jumping from the upper storeys of high-rise apartments has become the most popular method of committing suicide! Could any or all of these changes be justifiably attributed to industrialization? If so, to what extent? If we ask ourselves whether industrialization has made people happier or not, we also run into the difficulty of defining and quantifying what we mean by 'happiness'. We lack a generally acceptable 'happiness' index, or sufficiently sensitive indicators of social advancement. Moreover, what may be accepted to be indicators of progress or prosperity by some may be construed as pointers towards a sick society by others.

CONCLUSION

The word 'conclusion' is perhaps a misnomer, because the whole of my paper is based on the premise that while we can see momentous changes taking place in South-East Asia and the direct effects of industrialization on the health of workers, we are not yet in a position to evaluate quantitatively either the benefit or harm of industrialization or to balance the one against the other.

We maintain, nonetheless, that South-East Asia offers a unique opportunity to study the social and health effects of industrialization, even though we may not know exactly what they are. Some of the changes which occurred during the hundred and fifty years of the Industrial Revolution in the West are being re-enacted over decades in South-East Asia. The South-East Asia Ministers of Education Organization has set up a Tropical Medicine and Public Health programme, in an attempt to pool the scanty training and research resources in the region. Singapore has been selected as its centre for the study of Urban Health and Occupational Medicine.

It is hoped that in the next few years or so we shall be able to gather more knowledge and arrive at more concrete conclusions about the impact of industrial growth on health in South-East Asia. It may be, of course, that we shall never have the whole picture, but it is surely a worthwhile goal to advance the frontiers of knowledge about this most important subject. We can at least take consolation from the words of John Bowlby: 'It must be remembered that evidence is never complete, that knowledge of truth is always partial and that to seek certainty is to await eternity'.

ACKNOWLEDGEMENTS

I thank Dr Ang Swee Chai for help in the preparation of this paper and Miss Helen Chung for her clerical assistance.

Discussion

Ashby: Who makes the machines that have no safety devices, Professor Phoon?

Phoon: I wouldn't single out any particular country, but certainly many machines coming from developed countries do not have guards.

Ashby: So some of the faults lies in our exporting what is really evil material.

Dickinson: The guards would be available, but would not necessarily be sent with the machine unless asked for.

Mars: Very often if the guards are sent, they are removed in the factories.

Phoon: That does happen. We find instances of workers paid by piece work who, in attempting to speed up their rate of working, remove the guards and get their fingers chopped off.

Challis: What Professor Phoon's paper brings out, including the case of the girl injured by a circular saw, is that people are people, the world over. In every country, workers remove the guards from machinery, and it is no use condemning the worker. I hold as a very strong tenet that it is management's responsibility to ensure that people are protected from their own foolishness. It's not very useful to say 'That's a stupid man; he ought to have realized'. The only way to get people not to behave stupidly (and I wonder if this is being done in Singapore), is by turning to the modern tools of the mass media, and running an education programme. I don't mean lectures and school rooms, but using the mass media in the way they are used to sell soap flakes. In other words, you put up posters, you run film clips on television, which emphasize how serious it is to cut your fingers off. Even in developed countries that sort of campaign can have beneficial results. My second point is that when you do run campaigns like this you increase the pressure on the management side of industry to carry out their responsibilities, both legal and moral. So you should not be surprised to find some management reaction against such campaigns, particularly if run by a centralized civic community body. Managers are people too: nobody likes to be needled about his competence to run the job! My point is that in looking at industrial safety one must bear in mind that workers have to be educated in simple things and one has to drive home the moral responsibility of management to provide and continue to insist on the use of safety precautions. Finally, it must be remembered that as you go up the ladder of technology, the *hidden* dangers can become greater. It is easy to see a guard absent from a guillotine; it is not easy to see the absence of quality of technical management. Both chemical processing, and the materials processed, if released or upset, can be just as dangerous to a worker or to the community as can a guillotine that chops off fingers.

Jones: I would disagree with your optimism over the use of the mass media, and I will be discussing that in more detail in my paper (pp. 203–209). But I agree that one can find primitive working conditions in London just as in Singapore, and I think human nature is probably similar if not identical in this respect. I don't think it's a function of overdevelopment or underdevelopment. Environmental conditions of this type are caused by man himself. Perhaps it is a function of the smaller factory that man's nature is allowed to flower in small groups!

I am not so concerned about the effects of that sort of small factory on the total impact of cases of disease, because, as Dr Gilson mentioned, the total number affected in relation to the overall national burden of industrially induced mortality and morbidity is relatively small. But I am concerned with the use of the work place as a focus for the delivery of medical care. In Singapore, as we have heard, the focus of the delivery of medical care is the hospital or the private practitioner, and in an urban environment is therefore readily available. But in more scattered and less urbanized communities, with less developed systems of medical care, it is possible to use developing industry, no matter the size of unit, as a springboard and focus for developing a national system of medical care, rather than, as is traditional in western countries, using the family. In fact Eastern European countries have done just this and claim an adequate system of medical care equal to ours and by our standards.

Papanek: Minimally, three stances seem possible regarding work safety. One would be the loose *laissez faire* attitude illustrated by Professor Phoon. The second, most common in the US, Japan, the UK and parts of Western Europe, is to provide some work safety devices in a somewhat paternalistic way by the government, the industry or both. The third, which I find most appealing, is one being used in Denmark and Sweden. Here determination of work safety rests in the hands of the workers. As soon as it is felt that workers need ear protectors the process causing too much noise is examined. Workers don't like wearing ear protectors because they are uncomfortable, sweaty and moreover dangerous in isolating workers from sounds and instructions. Hence the corporation doesn't spend time and money on a routine con job, trying to convince workers that they ought to wear protective devices for their own good. Instead, the work process is discontinued until it has been made quiet enough so that ear protectors are no longer required.

In 1972 some of you may have suffered with me through a shortage of Danish Beer. This happened because the bottling plants were closed for over half a year until the company could make the process of bottle-making quiet enough to do away with ear protectors (except in a few isolated cases). One of my graduate students is working witht the TUC in Great Britain to design decibel level diagnostic devices as well as pollution level diagnostic devices to be used by trade union members in negotiating realistic working conditions. This would eliminate the inequality now existing where, because of differing work safety standards, foreseeably three in one hundred workers manufacturing polyvinyl chloride plastics in the UK will die of cancer of the liver during the next ten years, whereas in Germany and the US this death rate has now been reduced to nil.

Dickinson: Professor Phoon described some apparently dangerous situations, but I don't find them so horrific. This is because it is obvious what the dangers are and, in the subculture of industry, you may demonstrate your manhood by ritual exposure to known hazards. When I was an apprentice in British industry you took the guards off to show you were as tough as the next man. In Latin America, *machismo* demands that you should not have such things in the way, and that you should take the risks. If you work in an iron foundry you work in bare feet to show you are in perfect control. This is part of a society where people have their own social structure and status, which the outside inspector can never understand, and changes are only likely to come about by a collective decision to use the protective devices. In this way no one loses his status by being the first to adopt, say, safety goggles. This is a sociological problem that is unlikely to be modified greatly by distant legislation. I see little difference between *machismo* in Latin America and what happened in the factory in Chelmsford where I was an apprentice.

El Batawi: I agree that the workers themselves may sometimes remove the machine guards, but I don't think this is the main reason for the absence of safety devices in many work establishments. Dangerous machinery is sometimes imported to developing countries because many of the industries there are operated by multinational corporations, or by foreign firms, who may send them cheap machinery, and no servicing, and try to use cheap labour. I have seen factories in Hong Kong, Pakistan, Burma, Indonesia and other countries that are operated by foreign enterprises which use imported, old, worn-out machinery, and these have too many hazards. Absence of safety devices may also be the fault of the employers themselves. Sophisticated machinery is more expensive and they bring used machines from other industrial countries which are automating their processes and are therefore getting rid of old-fashioned and usually hazardous machinery.

Porter: Purchasing second-hand machinery may or may not be a sensible thing to do but it does not follow that machinery that has become obsolete in a highly developed industrial society, simply because of technical change, and may be perfectly suitable for a different state of industrialization, is therefore unsafe. One shouldn't label all second-hand machinery as unsafe machinery.

I would like also to know the evidence that the standards of safety in factories or industrial enterprises operated by multinational corporations in overseas countries are less than the standards adopted there by local employers. Professor Phoon's illustrations were not of multinational corporations but of conditions in small-scale industries. It is in fact argued that the multinational corporation commits the opposite crime in that it pays higher wages and has rather better standards of industrial practice than other local enterprises, and brings up wages to uneconomical levels.

Dickinson: I take Dr El Batawi's point, but when interlocks are put on machines, one of the ways people strike back, to prove they are still human in an impersonal industrial situation, is to show they understand the machine well enough to fool it. The imagination and ingenuity that goes into this is very real: it is the individual holding out against the alien system and though it appears misguided I believe it to represent creativity at a high level. The only way to solve such problems of industrial safety is to realize that safety measures are adopted only when people have positive reasons for wishing to be safe. Such a desire will come only from reasons that are valid in their own subculture of the shop floor and will be little influenced by academic armchair reasoning.

Second-hand machinery and safety are not directly connected, but the idea persists that there is something wrong with using such equipment. In the United States, two-thirds of all engineering production is thought to be on second-hand machines. If you have a cost-plus contract with the government you buy, every year, new machines of the most sophisticated type available, then sell them through your broker, at the end of the year, and somebody else picks them up and uses them. Regular chains have been established, up to thirteenth hand, where the machinery starts in a sophisticated industry, works its way through to the West coast of the US, and the thirteenth broker puts it on a ship for Taiwan. These chains exist elsewhere. Textile machinery taken as reparations by the USSR from West Germany at the end of the war was used in Russia to help re-establish their industry. Later it was refurbished and then passed on to China where it was modified and improved during use and then sent to a textile factory in Tanzania. When skills are developed, and better machinery is adopted in Tanzania, it is already booked to go on to the Somali Republic. The establishment of such chains has a lot to do with the rational use of means of production and with keeping capital costs down. Once this is ritualized and supplemented by the transfer of skills the transfer of concern for safety will be through the human rather than the mechanical elements of the chain. I believe we are doing a disservice to the process of development if we persist in suggesting that it is valid to assume that the second-hand is inherently unsafe.

Murray: I am also interested in the point that obviously people in Singapore, whether management or workers, behave like people anywhere else; but the odd thing is, that although people as individuals can be ingenious in defying the interlock on guards, or so careless or thoughtless, either as management or workers, that they produce injuries, nevertheless people have a collective conscience. On the subject of unguarded machines, there is an international collective conscience in the shape of the convention of the International Labour Organization on the prevention of the sale and hire of unguarded machinery. I wonder, Professor Phoon, how the collective conscience works in Singapore or in South-East Asia, as regards workers and their attitude towards safety? Although individual workers may be careless or ingenious and all the other things that human beings are, is any collective effort being made by trade unions to deal with the prevention of accidents and disease in industry in your area?

Phoon: The National Trades Union Congress of Singapore is very conscious of the need for safety and good health and has set up an Occupational Health and Safety Committee which has been trying to educate trade unionists about the importance of health and safety; they have also pressed the government to introduce more measures on such matters. The collective conscience, certainly among the more enlightened industrialists, and also among many trade unionists, has been good, but a large segment of the working population is not yet unionized—not that the trade unions are not pressing for better safety standards in general, but such people are more out of reach of the health education programmes of the unions.

I agree entirely on the hidden or chemical hazards. In fact a lecture I gave recently to the trade unions was called 'the Unseen Enemies': in other words, you can see the mechanical hazards but the chemical or carcinogenic hazards are just as real although not so visible. We have been trying to use the mass media for health education programmes. There have been campaigns; there has been a mobile exhibition to warn workers in the granite quarries about the danger of silicosis, and this is making some impact, although we sometimes feel that we are merely preaching to the converted. When we hold campaigns, people who are already aware of the dangers come but the small factory managers can't afford to do so, because they are also the clerk, the accountant, and so on and can't leave their jobs. The only way is for us to go to them, rather than expect them to come to us.

While it is true that there are few machine guards which cannot be removed and which will beat people's ingenuity, we should still persevere in insisting on proper guards because injuries from machines can be so very serious or even fatal.

References

1. MYRDAL, G. (1968) *Asian Drama*, vol. 2, p. 1150, Allen Lane, The Penguin Press, London
2. FEDERATION OF MALAYA (1963) Second Five-Year Plan, quoted in *Interim Review of Development in Malaya under the Second Five-Year Plan, Malaya*, p. 43
3. FEDERATION OF MALAYA (1957) *Report of the Industrial Development Working Party*, p. 4
4. YEH, S. H. K. (1971) Trends and issues in social development. In *The Singapore Economy* (You, P. S. & Lim, C. Y., eds.), p. 266, Eastern Universities Press, Singapore
5. Ref. 4, p. 272
6. PHOON, W. O. (1971) *Health and Safety at Work*, p. 21, National Safety First Council of Singapore, Singapore
7. EL BATAWI, M. A. (1968) The need for developing occupational health and safety programmes in relation to industrialization in Asia and the Far East. *Singapore Medical Journal 9*, 220
8. WORLD ASSEMBLY OF YOUTH (1967) *Youth and Urbanization in Asia*, p. 132, World Assembly of Youth, Belgium
9. WORLD HEALTH ORGANIZATION (1971) *Report of Inter-regional Seminar on Training and Services in Occupational Health for Developing Countries*, Indonesia, p. 3
10. BAKACS, T. (1972) *Urbanization and Human Health*, pp. 51-52, Akademiai Kiado, Budapest
11. JEGASOTHY, S. J. (1967) The social impact of urbanization. In *WAY Asian Seminar on Urbanization*, p. 25, Singapore
12. REDDY, K. V. (1967) An unfinished revolution. In *Youth and Urbanization in Asia*, p. 104, World Assembly of Youth, Belgium
13. ROBLESS, C. L. (1968) Malaysian agriculture and economic development. In *The Mission of Agriculture*, p. 2, Malaysian Centre for Development Studies, Prime Minister's Department, Kuala Lumpur
14. WASSERMANN, M. (1968) Problems of toxicology in industry and agriculture in developing countries. *Proceedings of the Lagos International Seminar on Occupational Health for Developing Countries*, p. 129, Lagos
15. VELLA, F. & PHOON, W. O. (1959) A clinical case of 6-glucose-phosphate dehydrogenase deficiency. *Medical Journal of Malaya 13*, 309-312
16. NGUYEN, DANG QUE (1972) Occupational health and safety in small industries in Vietnam. In *Proceedings of the 1st Symposium on Occupational Health in S.E. Asia*, Singapore, pp. 84-86
17. WONGPANICH, M., KRITALUGSANA, S. & DEEMA, P. (1972) Survey of pesticide hazards in agriculture. In *Proceedings of the 1st Symposium on Occupational Health in S.E. Asia*, Singapore, pp. 185-188
18. TRISHNANANDA, M. & ATTANATHO, V. (1972) Some observations on lead poisoning in Thailand. In *Proceedings of the 1st Symposium on Occupational Health in S.E. Asia*, Singapore, pp. 182-184
19. Ref. 9, p. 28
20. SUMA'MUR, P. K. (1972) Occupational health and national development. In *Proceedings of the 1st Symposium on Occupational Health in S.E. Asia*, Singapore, pp. 5-8
21. Ref. 9, p. 16
22. UNITED NATIONS ORGANIZATION (1966) *Industrial Development*, vol. III, p. 14, United Nations, New York
23. Ref. 9, p. 23
24. HUAN, S. H. (1971) Measures to promote industrialization. In *The Singapore Economy* (You, P. S. & Lim, C. Y., eds.), p. 243, Eastern Universities Press, Singapore
25. GOH, C. T. (1969) Industrial growth, 1959-66. In *Modern Singapore* (Ooi, J. B. & Chiang, H. D., eds.), p. 128, University of Singapore Press, Singapore
26. PHOON, W. O. (1975) Safety and health in Singapore. *Proceedings of the 7th World Congress on the Prevention of Occupational Accidents and Diseases*, Dublin, May 1974, in press

27. INDUSTRIAL HEALTH UNIT (1972) *Annual Report*, pp. 32-33, Ministry of Labour, Singapore
28. PHOON, W. O. (1973) Occupational health problems in urban Singapore. In *Science and the Urban Environment in the Tropics (Proceedings of the 2nd Congress of the Singapore National Academy of Science)*, pp. 62-68, Singapore
29. PHOON, W. O. & ALFRED, E. R. (1965) A study of stonefish (*Synanceja*) stings in Singapore with a review of the venomous fishes in Malaysia. *Singapore Medical Journal 6*, 158-163
30. PHOON, W. O., CHEW, P. K., TAN, S. B., WONG, H. K. C. & PHOON, W. H. (1974) A survey of health conditions in small factories in Singapore. In *Proceedings of the 9th Malaysia-Singapore Congress of Medicine*, in press
31. *Occupational Health in Japan, Proceedings of the XVIth International Congress on Occupational Health*, Tokyo (1969) pp. 189-190
32. PHOON, W. O. (1969) Factors impeding the progress of occupational health in a developing country. In *Proceedings of the XVIth International Congress on Occupational Health*, Tokyo, pp. 280-282
33. *Straits Times* (1974) August 28th, Singapore

Japanese experience on health and industrial growth

H. SAKABE

In Japan, industrial growth of the western type began in 1868, after the fall of the feudal system. The new central government directed its policy toward 'the wealth and armament of the country'. For this purpose, an increase in production was thought to be of major importance. The new government did away with the class distinctions between warriors, farmers, artisans and tradesmen of the feudal age and allowed people the freedom to choose their own jobs. It removed restrictions on domestic and overseas travel, and allowed people to choose where they lived, and to own property. These measures established the basis for freedom of economic activity. Finally, the government introduced economic systems and industries in the western style.

INDUSTRIAL GROWTH AND WORKERS' HEALTH

The first phase of industrial development was in transportation, including railways and shipping, and in mining. The second phase took place in the textile industry. Limited capital and an abundant labour force stimulated the growth of the textile industry.

Conditions as miserable as those of the workers in the Industrial Revolution in England were also experienced in Japan from about 1898 to 1918. In particular, serious occupational health hazards were encountered by those working in the mining and textile industries. In the former, workers suffered from silicosis and in the latter, from poor labour conditions and an inadequate work environment which led to a high mortality from tuberculosis in young women workers.

A few Japanese were aware that England had passed a number of factory acts during the 19th century and that the health of workers should be protected by legislation and inspection, but they were too weak during this period to

127

arouse public opinion. However, in 1916 the Factory Law went into effect in Japan.

During the Second World War the increasing production of war supplies took place in harmful environments and under severe labour conditions, and we still see the impact of this period on health. In 1972, for example, 37 cases of lung cancer were found in people who had worked in a copper-refining factory during the Second World War.

Since 1945 expansion has been rapid in all fields of industry in Japan, especially the heavy industries such as iron and steel, the machine industry, the motor industry and shipbuilding, and the heavy chemical industry. Industrial growth was so rapid that the product of mining and industry in 1970 was about 36 times as large as in 1947, and the annual average rate of growth of the Gross National Product (GNP) has been about 10% from about 1950. The Labour Standard Law, which made great advances on the Factory Law, was enacted in 1947 in order that the fundamental human rights of workers should be secured. This law, which deals with workers' health problems, has been powerfully enforced by about 2500 labour standard inspection officers who are part of the Ministry of Labour and are distributed throughout the country. Many potential risks of health hazards produced by a high rate of industrial growth have been counteracted by these legal and administrative measures. Furthermore, in 1972 the Japanese Government established the Industrial Safety and Health Law, which corresponded to changing circumstances in industry.

INDUSTRIAL GROWTH AND HEALTH HAZARDS DUE TO ENVIRONMENTAL POLLUTION

Rapid industrial growth has produced severe environmental pollution, and effective counter-measures were not taken until about 1967. The main health hazards resulting from environmental pollution are described below (and see ref. 1).

Minamata disease on the coast of Minamata Bay

The first patient with Minamata disease was found in 1956, in Minamata City on the west coast of Kyushu Island. From medical records and conversation with the inhabitants the disease was shown to have existed from 1953, but its existence had been concealed, since it was assumed to be contagious. In 1959 it was concluded that Minamata disease was a disturbance of the central nervous system mainly due to poisoning by an organic mercury compound as a result of the eating of large amounts of sea food from the Minamata Bay and its vicinity. Mercury, used in the production of acetaldehyde in a chemical plant in Minamata city, had drained into the sea in the form of inorganic mercury compounds and methylmercury, and the former compounds were converted into alkylmercury compounds in fish, shellfish and other marine organisms. Up to the end of June 1974 patients numbered 784, including 96 deaths.

Minamata disease in the Agano River basin

In 1965 Minamata disease was again found, this time in villages along the Agano River in Niigata prefecture of Honshu Island. The cause here was the alkylmercury taken in by freshwater fish in the Agano River, which was polluted with mercury from a chemical factory along the river. The patients numbered 461, including 20 deaths, up to the end of June 1974.

Itai-Itai disease

Since about 1910 it had been noted that a strange disease of unknown origin had been endemic along the lower or middle reaches of the Jinzu River in the central part of the Japan Sea side of Honshu Island. Patients complained of severe pain and often cried out 'itai-itai' (ouch-ouch), and the inhabitants called the condition 'itai-itai disease'. At first it was assumed to be a nutritional disturbance but by 1967 many studies suggested that cadmium played a major role in its onset. Patients were mainly post-menopausal women living in areas heavily polluted with cadmium. Clinical findings included symptoms of senile osteomalacia and skeletal deformation. In particular, bone pain and convulsions of the femoral abductor muscles were intensified by movement. Low-molecular-weight protein and cadmium in the urine was also common. In this case, cadmium from a mining and refining factory had polluted the Jinzu river and the soil of rice paddies, and the inhabitants had absorbed cadmium from water and food. Up to the end of June 1974 patients numbered 125, including 50 deaths.

Respiratory disorders due to air pollution

Apart from these disasters resulting from polluted water, the numbers of patients with chronic respiratory disorders, including chronic bronchitis, bronchial asthma and emphysema, caused by urban air pollution, have increased in industrial cities such as Yokkaichi, Kawasaki and Osaka.

Hazards due to photochemical smog

From 1970, a new type of health hazard resulting from urban air pollution in summer has been noticed. Although most complaints have been of smarting eyes and throat irritation, some people have complained of serious symptoms such as difficulty in breathing, numbness of the limbs, or cramps. Serious attacks occur during or immediately after strenuous physical exercise outdoors. The pathogenesis is not clear. Since the patients are found only in summer, it is assumed that irritating or toxic substances are formed photochemically by the strong ultraviolet radiation of the sun in the polluted, hot and highly humid atmosphere. The reported cases, including those with mild symptoms only, numbered over 30 000 from 1970 to 1973 throughout Japan.

In face of such a serious environmental situation the Japanese Government has passed many laws for the prevention of environmental pollution since 1967, and established the Environmental Agency in 1971. But in general it may be said that Japan had failed in the prevention and control of the environmental pollution accompanying rapid industrial growth.

CHARACTERISTICS OF ENVIRONMENTAL POLLUTION AND ITS EFFECT IN JAPAN

Why has environmental pollution progressed to such a serious stage and why have specific diseases due to pollution, that have never been experienced in other countries, occurred in Japan?

Natural conditions

The amount of flat land in Japan is only 19.4% of the total land area, and of this 16.2% is tilled for agriculture and the remaining 3.2% is used for residential areas, factory sites and roads. Industrial development has mainly taken place in the hinterland of already established industrial cities or in the coastal areas. In the former, air pollution in each city has been increased. In the latter coastal areas, many heavy chemical industries which developed very rapidly after the war have been constructed mainly on reclaimed land along the Pacific Sea, with sea transportation in view. Since these plants have been built in close relation to each other, to facilitate the transport of materials, they form a compact belt of factories along the coast and have become powerful sources of water and air pollution. They have provoked respiratory disorders among the inhabitants of Yokkaichi and other cities by air pollution and have harmed fish by water pollution.

It is important to note that industrial growth in Japan has taken place within a very small area. A comparison of GNP per square kilometre of flat land shows that Japan has the highest rate among the industrial countries. The GNP per unit of flat land in Japan is 14 times as large as that of USA, 5 times that of France and Italy, 3.5 times that of the UK and 1.7 times that of West Germany[2]. It seems likely that, in general, the very rapid industrial growth in a small area with a high population density and without effective counter-measures against pollution has produced the present serious environmental pollution in Japan. The Japanese climate should not be overlooked as a contributory factor. The very hot and humid weather in summer may enable toxic substances to be formed in the urban air by a photochemical reaction, as already indicated.

Food

Rice and fish are the main Japanese foods. Carbohydrate is mainly supplied through rice and protein mainly through fish. Many Japanese like to eat coastal fish and also eat raw fish—a dietary habit rarely seen in western developed countries. Minamata disease had been caused by organic mercury compounds in coastal and freshwater fish, and has never been seen in countries which lack either pollution of water with mercury, or a diet in which fish-eating predominates.

Industrial technology in Japan

Industrialization was born and first developed in western countries, and its development was characterized by repeated trial and error. The 'error' aspect has been recognized not only from the standpoints of the economy and productivity, which are implicit in technology itself, but also from that of the effects on the environment. In 1892, A. E. Fletcher, Chief Alkali Inspector in the UK, in a lecture entitled 'Modern legislation in restraint of the emission of noxious gases from manufacturing operations', said:

'I think I am right, therefore, in saying that in this Act a new principle was thus introduced, one differing from that of simple repression, hitherto applied wherever an admitted evil of the kind was dealt with. There was herein an acknowledgement that with the evil there was associated a greater good, and that to sweep away the one would be to destroy the other; that it must suffice to restrain the evil, to insist on the adoption of the best practicable means for diminishing it to the furthest possible limit'.

Fletcher pointed out that some manufacturing operations were evil and described how to control that evil. In the developed countries, technology has been compelled to adapt to society, and society has also adapted to the technology. Japan has copied many industrial plants and processes developed in the West, and her technologists have tended to assume that imported techniques would be harmless in Japan, since no trouble had been experienced in developed countries. But in the field of industrial health, for example, we had the experience that spinning hands had difficulty working on the imported tall spinning machines, and we still have a similar health hazard in the operation of punching machines designed for westerners—a hazard that has not been experienced in the developed countries. These are problems of ergonomics, and relate to racial physical differences which enter into the working of the 'man–machine' system. Health hazards resulting from exposure to toxic substances in the factory have not differed greatly between the developed countries and Japan, on the other hand.

It seems that a factory is a relatively closed society without too many complicating factors, whereas the environment is an 'open' society organized by many factors which are closely linked with each other, and differ in different countries. The concept of an 'environment–industry' system may be useful for considering industrial technology in relation to environmental pollution, comparable to the idea of a 'man-machine' system in industry. The environment and the manufacturing process are inseparable, and the manufacturing process should be adapted to the environment. In this sense, Japanese industrial technologists ought to have considered how to adapt foreign industrial techniques to the characteristic environment of Japan.

Structural features of Japanese society

Social institutions in Japan have always been closed systems. Their organization has a characteristic structure in which the members are tied vertically into a graded, hierarchic order. Employees have been loyal to the companies to whom they belong, and companies have taken care of their living conditions and welfare until retirement and even after it. Nakane[3] has defined Japanese society as a vertical society. The very rapid industrial growth in Japan has been motivated by intense competition among companies. It can be said in general that industrial health has been the problem of industry, which is a 'vertical' society, while environmental health is a problem in the community, which is a 'horizontal' society. Our relative success in the former and failure in the latter perhaps originates from these structural features of Japanese society. Local authorities and the leaders of local communities have been conservative and have welcomed the establishment of new plants by companies because they expected that industrialization in their districts would improve their financial situation. Therefore, they could not protest firmly against environmental pollution from these plants. However, the three disasters described earlier, and the health hazards resulting from air pollution in Yokkaichi, provoked a strong movement by the inhabitants against environmental pollution, and this has grown rapidly. Public opinion, stimulated by the inhabitants' protests, has become very critical of the pollution.

The lack of counter-measures against pollution

The Japanese Government passed a Water Quality Conservation Law for the prevention of water pollution in 1958, and a Basic Law for Environmental Pollution Control which established the basic principle for the prevention of environmental pollution in 1967. In Japan, the problem of water pollution had become a sensitive area in which the interests of mining and industries and of farmers and fishermen have clashed. The law in 1958, which stressed this point, was not an effective counter-measure against water pollution. By 1967, when the Basic Law for Environmental Pollution Control was enacted, environmental pollution in Japan had already progressed very far, because although there had been many local complaints as a result of emission products from factories, no strong public opinion demanding powerful counter-measures had arisen until 1960.

GENERAL DISCUSSION

Prospective evaluation and early detection of health hazards

Since about 1960 the Japanese chemical industry has produced many new chemicals. Some have been used only in factories as raw materials in manufacturing processes; others have been brought into use in daily life. The extent of the use of new materials or commodities has been restricted in some cases but in others their use has become so widespread that it becomes difficult to withdraw these chemicals from human use even if they are proved to cause health hazards.

Recent experience with the manufacture of polyvinyl chloride illustrates this. Vinyl chloride vapour has been shown to cause haemangiosarcoma of the liver. In addition, hydrogen chloride gas, produced in the burning of waste material containing polyvinyl chloride, pollutes the air as well as destroying the furnaces. Nevertheless, to prohibit the manufacture and use of polyvinyl chloride would be almost impossible, since polyvinyl chloride products are now widely used in industry and in everyday life, because of the cheapness and usefulness of this material. The best way to prevent health hazards due to substances in industrial processes is clearly to investigate their toxicity *in advance* of their production, but our present stage of knowledge is not good enough for us to evaluate all potential hazards; and to make the necessary tests on all new chemical substances being used in industry would in any case be impossible. But animal experiments and other biological tests for toxicity to human beings should be planned on the substances to which many people are exposed or will be exposed. In the present situation, the early detection of new kinds of health hazard in workers and local inhabitants resulting from chemical substances is of vital importance, because it can prevent the further spread of the health hazard and minimize the number of victims.

Rate of industrial growth

A high industrial growth rate seems to fascinate statesmen, and has been used as a popular slogan as well. The rate of growth of GNP has stimulated economic competition between countries. If we consider it from the standpoint of its harmful secondary effects, however, the growth rate ought perhaps *not* to be so high, because the problems of health hazards and environmental pollution caused by industrial growth will take an extremely long time to resolve, requiring the evaluation of the hazard, the confirmation of the cause or causes, and the devising and implementing of preventive measures. If industrial growth continues to progress, leaving these problems unsolved, they may result in a disaster. In the past, capital, the labour force, natural resources, transportation and other factors have been the pacemakers of industrialization. The second-order effects of industrial growth should in the future also be an important pacemaker of industrial growth.

A basic question about industrial growth

Galbraith[4] has said that 'As a further consequence, goods that are related only to elementary physical sensation—that merely prevent hunger, protect against cold, provide shelter, suppress pain—have come to comprise a small and diminishing part of all production. Most goods serve needs that are discovered to the individual not by the palpable discomfort that accompanies deprivation, but by some psychic response to their possession. They give him a sense of personal achievement, accord him a feeling of equality with his neighbours, divert his mind from thought, serve sexual aspiration, promise social acceptability, enhance his subjective feeling of health, well-being or orderly peristalsis, contribute by conventional canons to personal beauty, or are otherwise psychologically rewarding'. And yet some of these goods have had a harmful effect on workers, have polluted the environment in the course of their manufacture, and have introduced problems in the disposal of their wastes. In addition, they have dissipated limited natural resources. If a cynical question is permitted, I should like to ask: what *is* industrial growth?

Discussion

Phoon: Dr Sakabe, what is the incidence of bladder cancer in Japan? A few years ago, when you had not yet banned the use of antioxidants like β-naphthylamine, whereas some western countries had already done so, I was told in Japan that a lot of new cases of bladder cancer were being found each year as a result of the use of such antioxidants. What measures are being taken to screen out people who are or were working in industries that used antioxidants in the past?

Sakabe: The Japanese Ministry of Labour has forbidden the production and use of β-naphthylamine and benzidine since 1972. People who had been exposed to these substances in their work carry registration books with them and receive a medical examination including urine tests, such as microscopic examination of sediments, and if necessary Papanicolaou's cell diagnosis, cystoscopy and other tests, twice a year.

Phoon: I also wonder about the situation with occupational dermatosis. In Singapore an increasing number of people suffer from it, as a result of various chemicals coming into contact with their skin during their work. We have done surveys in factories relating to engineering processes; cooling oils, for example, have given rise to a fairly high incidence of dermatosis. We had one instance of a factory, started by a developed country, which recruited young girls and sent them to that country to learn about the process. When they came back the workers discovered that they were under a legal bond to serve the company for up to four years. They found that they had to work in an oily atmosphere, and some of them developed disfiguring acneiform lesions which made female employees worried about their chances of marrying. Unfortunately, because of the legal bond, they had to work out their service, and in Singapore occupational dermatosis is not yet subject to compensation or notification.

Sakabe: We have no great trouble from occupational dermatosis, and almost no occupational skin cancer in Japan. This may be due to the fact that the Japanese bath a lot and place a lot of emphasis on personal hygiene, so they keep their skin in a relatively clean state.

Phoon: The Chinese and Japanese are very similar both ethnically and in terms of personal hygiene, so it is surprising that we have this increasing incidence of occupational dermatosis and you don't find it.

Sakabe: Occupational dermatosis has of course been observed in Japan, but it is not so troublesome a problem, as the work environment has been improved remarkably. In addition, there has been no unemployment in Japan and so workers could move freely, and if the sensitive worker suffered from dermatosis, he or she could move to another job.

Phoon: In Singapore we are short of labour, not jobs; but people who come from Malaysia seek jobs in Singapore and are under government contracts which require them not to change their job for three years. If they want to leave a job they have to go back to Malaysia, so in a sense they are under bond. This may explain the difference in incidence.

White: I want to take up the final paragraph of Dr Sakabe's paper where he expressed doubts about the wisdom of the Japanese pattern of development, and to point out that we have been hearing about the two countries, Singapore and Japan, with the highest income per head in Asia. I should like to broaden the discussion and orient it towards what I see as the main problems of the majority of undeveloped countries. This concerns the patterns of development they should seek, rather than simply how the environmental pollution created by a particular pattern of development affects the health of the population. In El Salvador, which I have visited and studied[5], I found that I could divide the provision of medical services into five levels (see Table 1).

The *top* level is that of private practice by people formally qualified in modern medicine, with a fee for service at a non-subsidized rate. At a guess, but one based on certain fragmentary statistics, 4% of the population are covered but 25% of the time of the country's doctors is spent on treatment within this sector.

The *second* level is that of the Salvadorean Social Security Institution together with small parallel services for certain government personnel. The total population is 4 million. The Social Security system covers only the 156 000 workers and employees of private businesses and 54 000 wives—that is, 5.3% of the people. The other parallel services, for government teachers, telecommunications workers, 'security forces', prisoners, and beneficiaries of rural colonization schemes, add in total another 2.0%. The Social Security Institution has an income, just for its health services, of 10% of the wage or salary of each person insured, and it amounted to £30 in 1974 for each person covered (children are not covered); this enables it to give, for instance, 4.1 consultations per

TABLE 1 (White)

Levels of health care in El Salvador

Level	% of population covered	Consultation payments made to doctors
1. Private practice (full fee)	4%	£1.30-£4.30
2. Social security etc.	7%	28p-45p
3. Ministry of Health (and charity)	35%	15p-30p
4. Practitioners without formal qualifications		
5. Traditional curers	54%	

Note: these percentages are of course rough indicators only, particularly in the sense that one person may well receive treatment at different levels on different occasions.

The payments made to doctors for consultation are converted into sterling at the rate of ₡5.80 per £1 (U.S.$2.32 per £1). They refer to 1974. The range at levels 1 and 2 is partly accounted for by the difference between specialist and non-specialist treatment; at level 3 it is almost entirely accounted for by the fact that the Ministry of Health currently pays its doctors in the capital almost double what it pays them in most provincial areas!

person covered, to maintain 3.2 hospital beds per 1000 covered, and to have money to spare. It also pays its doctors at a somewhat higher rate than the Ministry of Health.

The *third* level is that of the Ministry of Health, together with some private charitable institutions. The coverage of these charitable clinics is not a distinct population group—the same person might go to either for treatment—but to give a figure in terms of coverage, we might guess at another 4% or 5%, making the total coverage of modern medicine in the private sector 8% or 9%. The theoretical responsibility of the Ministry of Health is the other 85% of the population. For this it has a budget, per person theoretically covered, of £3.45. However, it might be more realistic to say that only a third of those theoretically covered are really covered, and that this third has £10 each per year of expenditure. This 'third' has to be vague, because it is a question of the distance which needs to be travelled to get to a health centre or post, and distances are not very great in El Salvador, so it cannot be said that anyone is entirely out of range; about a third are within five or six kilometres' distance.

The *fourth* level is that of modern medicine dispensed by people without formal qualifications and practising outside the formal institutions: practical nurses and dentists, unqualified chemists, and so on. They may of course have considerable practical knowledge and skill.

The *fifth* level is that of traditional medicine. In other countries the traditional curers might be subdivided further according to whether they belong to an Ayurvedic or similar formal school of written learning or whether their tradition is entirely oral. In El Salvador, the curers are all of this second type, although they too can be subdivided. Their numbers are large but entirely unknown because most of their treatment is illegal: they are, however, usually the only source of treatment outside the towns.

These levels correspond closely to levels of income, of those who have effective access to them, in the very unequal distribution of national income. They are levels of average expenditure per illness treated, including the expenditure on the education or training of those who do the treating, and in general a person has access to a certain level directly or indirectly according to his capacity to pay. A person who is ill has recourse, in general, to the most expensive (to provide) service to which he has access—that is to say, to the 'highest' of these levels; but for a more serious illness he may be disposed to pay above his normal capacity or to make a greater effort to obtain access to a service at a 'higher' level. Of course, some people prefer to be treated by someone they know personally at one of the two 'lowest' levels; then there are others, even doctors, who have recourse to 'empirical' or traditional remedies when the modern ones do them no good.

So far, we have concentrated in this symposium on an intervention at the second level, the level of social security, which is the level of employed people. Most of the discussion currently going on about how to give medical treatment, or preventive medicine, in the Third World, concentrates on the Ministry of Health level and is concerned to expand the effective coverage of its type of treatment, to cover more people lower down the scale. It seems to me that too little attention has been paid to a positive role of the practitioners operating at levels 4 and 5; they seem to be rejected, particularly those in the fifth section, as being merely an opposition to be overcome, for people to be weaned away from, rather than practitioners who are giving some sort of treatment. So far in the symposium we have not *even* discussed something as relatively worthwhile as the expansion of Ministry of Health services to the whole population. We have been discussing only what can be done about essentially a labour aristocracy —a group participating in the benefits of a kind of development which is not the sort that can benefit the whole population in these countries; because the kind of industry that provides employment for a certain small number of people can't be expanded, for lack of capital, to provide employment for everyone at the lower levels. We should be considering, therefore, whether it would not be sensible to compare, say, the cost of saving one life by providing safety devices on machines at the second level with the cost of saving one life by providing rural health clinics and providing some training for practitioners at the fifth level who are willing and able to give medical treatment, although they don't have much knowledge. If they were given more training, at a very much lower cost per life saved they could affect the problems of most of the population of the country.

Ashby: I like your scheme very much, but I think the reason we have concentrated on the second level is because we want to stick to the title of our symposium, which is 'Health and *Industrial* Growth'.

White: I was taking up Dr Sakabe's final point and suggesting that we should also be discussing the *type* of industrial growth, and whether the whole pattern of industrial growth being adopted in most developing countries is the correct pattern that will be most helpful to the population.

Illich: The difficulty, as I see it, is precisely that we succeed in pushing a few demonstration individuals from the fifth level up to the second level in Table 1 and thereby create the impression that the lower groups participate in this programme, when we can demonstrate, even on the third level, that the cost per head of the typical treatment for which this level is necessary is far beyond what could be provided for the overwhelming majority of the population, having the conditions for which this kind of treatment is prescribed.

Ramalingaswami: The situation in El Salvador fits well with the Indian scene too! Only the proportions may be different. There is a vast rural population engaged in agriculture, amounting to 125 million according to the 1971 Census, to the majority of whom modern health care is not readily accessible. It is this group that the government, through the Ministry of Health and through various health and welfare programmes, tries to reach, but because of a spread of health care from the top to the bottom, rather than building from the bottom upwards, and because of a system that has not taken enough care of the various factors that enable it to penetrate to the business end of health care delivery, it fails. It fails because the primary health centre, which should subserve the basic health needs of a population of 90–100 000 people, is rarely able to provide services to beyond a radius of three miles. The bulk of the population is left to be taken care of by practitioners and healers at levels 4 and 5. The amount of money that is actually being spent on taking care of the health of this population is extremely small per head, as Ivan Illich says, compared to the organized group at level 2. Possibly about six million people are involved in manufacturing household industry, and less than a million in the mining and quarrying industry. This is the kind of distortion we have.

References

1. ENVIRONMENTAL AGENCY (1972) *Pollution Related Diseases and Relief Measures in Japan*, Printing Bureau, the Japanese Ministry of Finance, Tokyo
2. FOOD AND AGRICULTURE ORGANIZATION (1971) *Production Year Book*, FAO, Rome
3. NAKANE, C. (1973) *Japanese Society*, Penguin Books, Middlesex
4. GALBRAITH, J. K. (1968) *The New Industrial State*, Hamish Hamilton, London
5. WHITE, A. (1973) *El Salvador*, pp. 239-243, Ernest Benn, London & Tonbridge, and Praeger, New York & Washington D.C.

Health of working populations in industrializing societies

M. A. EL BATAWI

The working populations in the less developed countries of Africa, Asia, Latin America, and Oceania are estimated to comprise 40% of the total population[1]. In the more industrially developed countries of Europe, North America and elsewhere they number almost 50%[1]. As workers are the main breadwinners and the backbone of economic and social progress, their health is an essential factor in development and represents an important human welfare goal. On the other hand, it has often been observed that they represent a risk group, especially in countries undergoing rapid industrialization. The risks are: (1) the rapid introduction of new work processes and technology unfamiliar to them, with the changes in their way of life and the stresses it entails; (2) the possible aggravation of highly prevailing ill-health by environmental work hazards and the weakness or absence of medical screening and environmental control; (3) the indiscriminate employment of vulnerable groups such as the young, the aged, and the partially handicapped in jobs that are not suited to their physical and mental capabilities; and (4) the uprooting of people from their original habitat and their migration to industrial areas or countries which are often associated with significant health and safety risks.

It seems therefore that health programmes in developing countries will have to take account of these new dimensions as early as possible, in addition to dealing with the general health problems that may be encountered with industrialization.

OBJECTIVES

This paper has two main objectives:

1. To describe in general terms the major health problems of the working populations in countries undergoing industrial development and the services available to them;

2. To review some of the policy lines in developing occupational health programmes and cite a few examples of approaches followed by different countries.

CONDITIONS OF HEALTH OF WORKERS

It is obvious that the specific health problems of workers vary geographically and in the different trades within geographic areas. The major health problems do not necessarily originate from work hazards, although they may be aggravated by the work environment.

General health problems

Overall environmental conditions play a great role in community health problems, which also affect workers, and the 'biological pollution' of the environment in developing countries, where disease-transmitting vectors and contaminated food and water are major factors of ill-health, is obviously more important than the pollution of the air by toxic by-products.

Communicable and parasitic diseases are still the major health problems of workers in these countries, in addition to malnutrition which increases vulnerability to disease both occupational and non-occupational. In those parts of the world where malnutrition exists, work output is poor and human susceptibility to further disability is high.

Parasitic infestation prevails particularly among agricultural workers and workers in the small industries, and in the absence of medical supervision it may also affect workers in large factories even though they may be economically better off[2].

Pulmonary tuberculosis was found in some countries to be more frequent among industrial workers than among the general population[3].

Occupational diseases

As regards occupational diseases, there has been inadequate systematic reporting, and the information available is mainly based on field investigations in developing countries. In many instances, these diseases constitute a major health problem, particularly with respect to the causation of permanent disability. In industry, poisoning by toxic substances is frequent. Respiratory irritants such as nitrogen oxides and acrolene result in a high incidence of acute respiratory disease and in chronic obstructive pulmonary disease from prolonged exposure[4]. Intoxication by heavy metals also occurs and some reports show a prevalence of up to 32% of lead absorption among exposed workers, and poisoning in a considerable proportion of those in lead smelting and battery manufacturing enterprises and in foundries[5].

The problem of the inhalation of organic and other vegetable dusts, causing respiratory allergy, asthma, chronic bronchitis, and other infections, is a major one. Occupational obstructive respiratory diseases and byssinosis occur in up to 58% of workers employed in cotton and flax[6], and silicosis has recently been reported in one country to occur among 12% of the workers examined in stone-crushing plants[7].

Occupational dermatosis remains one of the most common of occupational diseases, affecting in certain instances up to one-third of the workers exposed to mineral oils, cement and other substances.

Cancer-producing physical and chemical agents remain uncontrolled in workplaces in developing and industrial countries alike. The recent episode of cancer resulting from exposure to vinyl chloride in the plastic and rubber industry is an example pointing not only to the inadequacies of information on the carcinogenicity of industrial substances but also to the inadequacy of control measures and criteria.

In mining, pneumoconiosis remains an unsolved problem. This can be illustrated by the very high rate of payment of workmen's compensation benefits in several countries for the permanent disability caused by fibrotic diseases of the lung, resulting from the inhalation of different types of dusts. Miners originally affected by pulmonary tuberculosis are likely to acquire fibrogenic changes in the lungs in a short period of time. Mine accidents are one of the main causes of death in this sector of the working population.

In agriculture, infectious, parasitic and zoonotic diseases, and the increased use of agricultural chemicals including toxic pesticides, and the mechanization of agriculture with the high risk of accidental injury, are problems of increasing magnitude. Investigations made in one African country have shown the occurrence of ill-health resulting from exposure to organo-chlorine and organo-phosphorus compounds among 85% of the workers exposed[8]. Carcinogenic ulceration of varicose veins in female workers in the coffee plantations in one of these countries has resulted from exposure to arsenical pesticides[9].

In other trades, an example may be cited of transport workers, where road accidents inflict a high toll of mortality and disability every year. Workers on board ships and seafarers were found to be affected by a wide variety of communicable diseases, such as tuberculosis, venereal disease, and dysentery. They are not only victims of these diseases, but also carriers of the disease from one part of the world to another. The type of work they do is characterized by unusual psychosocial distress, with lack of identification with a home and of stability of life. In recent epidemiological studies, psychosomatic diseases like peptic ulcer were found to be significantly higher among seafarers than other groups, in addition to drug addiction and alcoholism.

Psychosocial factors at work

To a large extent, workers in the developing countries have managed to adapt to the new psychosocial environment of mechanized work. The benefits expected, mainly from material rewards and better pay, play an important role in motivation to meet new psychosocial challenges in industry that often involve psychological isolation, limited identification, and repetitive tasks. In many instances, however, adaptation may fail, either because of too much stress or personal susceptibility or both, resulting in desertion of work and bouts of high labour turnover and absenteeism or in psychological and psychosomatic disorder. Migrant workers face even more variables to which they must adapt, and up to now, only limited efforts have been directed to the health of migrants.

It should be emphasized, however, that work, when it is suitably adapted to human capacities and successfully enables human ambitions to be achieved, is an important factor in the promotion of health and should therefore be exploited to this end.

The problem of small industries

Small industries (employing under 50 workers) constitute a major sector of the total work force, particularly in developing countries. They are comparatively very numerous and they can hardly benefit from health inspection services. On their own, they often have no regular health services, while frequently suffering from inadequate environmental and health conditions. Because of economic factors, industrial development in the less developed countries relies more on the establishment of small factories than on large ones. Unless provision is made for adequate planning, the health problems of this large sector of the working population will remain unsolved. An approach relying mostly on the extension of public health services to these workplaces is essential.

Employment problems and workers' health

In some developing countries, the problem of overpopulation has repercussions on employment and on occupational health practice. Employers' motivation to implement occupational health programmes is in many instances reduced because of the many demands for the relatively few job opportunities. Underemployment reduces the economic value of workers, and it has also been associated with increased absenteeism from work and lower productivity.

Health services available to workers in industrializing countries

Because of the historical development of public health in industrializing countries, occupational health programmes have received scant attention. In certain cases these programmes are inadequate, poor, or non-existent. In some countries the role of health services has been ill-defined and limited to curative or palliative services to workers that are largely ineffective. In those countries, health or labour inspectors attempt to enforce laws dating back to colonial times and the enforcement machinery is often weak and untrained. General health programmes for workers in industry, including such programmes as the control of tuberculosis and other infectious diseases, nutrition and health education, are seldom developed.

The difficulties seem to have evolved from several factors, including mainly the historical inheritance of inadequate programmes, the lack of experience in occupational health, the absence of adequate information on the health problems of workers and their magnitude, the absence of guiding principles in establishing occupational health programmes within the framework of public health services, and the classical difficulties in coordination between the different governmental departments concerned with workers' health.

POLICY LINES IN OCCUPATIONAL HEALTH PROGRAMMING

The need

The paramount objective of any society is the welfare of its people and the improvement of the quality of life. All other factors, such as economic resources, industry, mineral wealth, and agriculture, are only of value insofar as they help attain this objective. It is therefore obvious that health, defined as a state of complete physical, mental, and social well-being, is a major component of the main objective of nations.

Countries undergoing development have often suffered the striking effects of poverty and disease, and are coming to learn that these can only be tackled by a coordinated attack on all the causative elements, that are to a great extent interdependent. If the causes of the ills of developing societies are interdependent, so should be the measures to combat these ills. Health programmes have therefore to be closely coordinated with all other measures to combat poverty by economic and industrial development and by social enlightenment and education. On the other hand, societies should not be carried away by the luring attraction of wealth through industrialization and the mounting figures of production of material elements, forgetting in the process their main purpose, which is the human being, and his health and welfare. More precisely they should not allow industry, production and work to be a source of illness, handicap and disability among their people, as is so often found.

It is mainly for these reasons that labour protective legislation was enacted at some stage of the Industrial Revolution in Western Europe, and that this finally evolved into the development of occupational health and safety and workers' compensation laws.

In addition, the whole field of occupational health, with its preventive medical and environmental hygiene components, emerged as a public health discipline with a large body of knowledge and research on the interaction between man and his work environment, the effects on health of hazardous exposures, the mechanism of action of toxic agents, the early detection of disease, environmental evaluation and control, and the humanization of working life.

Insofar as occupational health and safety laws are concerned, there is no doubt in my mind that these are necessary, provided there is a reasonably effective machinery for implementing them. In my experience, however, legislation cannot on its own be the only or even the major means by which governments try to achieve their occupational health objectives. There should always be the essential components relating to human nature and performance in the building-up of human conscience, understanding, and cooperation, which will lead to the honest assessment of needs, the creation and development of effective preventive health services, and the keen interest in extending these to all those incapable of establishing them on their own. Whether this should be stimulated by education and training or by demonstrating the economic value of a healthy worker, or both, they are undoubtedly as important as, or even more important than legislation and enforcement, and to a large extent more lasting and effective.

The totality of health

The simple logic in developing occupational health services indicates that a comprehensive approach to the total health problems of the workers should be adopted. Workers are people affected by general diseases in addition to occupational risks. They are an integral part of the community, and it makes little sense to see occupational health services in isolation from community health programmes. Furthermore, the industrializing countries cannot afford duplication or fragmentation of effort. With the limited resources available to them, a serious attempt should be made to utilize these resources in the most effective manner, and in this sense the health personnel providing services to workers in factories, mines, and organized agriculture should carry out a comprehensive preventive health programme to the workers and their families. On the other hand, governmental public health officers should extend preventive health measures to workplaces and make use of the convenience in dealing with a population that is easily reached and whose health can systematically be monitored and evaluated, and where the effectiveness of control measures can immediately be demonstrated.

Occupational health therefore plays an important role in public health. Indeed, it is about the only field of public health where most of the elements relating to environment and man can systematically and effectively be dealt with and quantitatively evaluated.

EXAMPLES OF MODERN APPROACHES TO OCCUPATIONAL HEALTH IN DEVELOPING COUNTRIES

By way of conclusion, I should like to refer to a number of examples of modern occupational health programmes in some industrializing countries that can be considered as guides toward the solution of the health problems of workers.

1. The development of occupational health within the framework of national health services

In Thailand, the Sudan and other countries, the national health services have recently established comprehensive programmes of occupational health that carry out environmental evaluation and control of occupational hazards, periodic medical examination of workers by health centres established with the employers' participation, control of communicable diseases and malnutrition in industry, and care of illness and injuries. These are closely coordinated with inspection of workplaces and enforcement of legislation. These programmes also investigate different health problems resulting from different hazardous exposures in industry.

2. The development of occupational health services for small industries

In the Republic of Korea, Singapore and other countries, several programmes dealing with the health problems of workers in small industries have recently been developed. The main features of these programmes are:

(a) the extension of governmental industrial health services to small industries;

(b) the development of inter-enterprise cooperative schemes of health services with governmental and private professional support.

3. *The use of occupational health manpower in comprehensive national programmes*

In Burma and other countries, occupational health workers have recently been required to bring comprehensive preventive health services to workers and their families. This is expected substantially to promote national health services and to improve national health statistics. Similar models are being planned in Guinea and other countries.

I have great hopes of the promising future in developing adequate health programmes for working people in industrializing countries that will avoid the mistakes of earlier industrial movements and deal with both the problems prevailing and those foreseen in this rapidly changing human society. Industry should not be regarded as an evil or a menace to the tranquil agricultural communities of the Third World. It is a way of economic progress and its risks are preventable. The man-made environment of work, with its sophisticated technology, can still be controlled by intelligent and wise endeavour.

Discussion

Phoon: Dr El Batawi made the important point that in addition to the physical hazards of the environment there are psychological hazards. We have had many problems of this kind. As an example, in a South-East Asian country an attempt was made, when that country was gaining independence, to hand over some responsibility to local people. Young men were recruited and groomed to succeed expatriates. Some of these men were intelligent but lacked experience and developed psychological problems because of feelings of inadequacy. I was called in to study the differential sickness-absenteeism rates between four shifts of workers whose ethnic composition was about the same; they were engaged in the same process, in the same factory. But the sickness-absenteeism rate of one shift was much greater than those of the other three. We found that the main reason for this high rate was not physical sickness but poor morale, which was in turn due to a lack of confidence in the shift leader, who was very young and feeling very insecure. His insecurity transmitted itself to the people working under him. It is well known that psychological problems are just as 'infectious' as measles or whooping cough: they can be transmitted from one person to another. In this case, the man was given further training and moral support and later the sickness rate of his shift went down.

In another incident, a man who was well-esteemed by his superiors and colleagues came to me weeping. He was afraid that something would go wrong while he was in charge. Actually, everybody had confidence in him; he was competent and efficient, but he could not overcome his feelings of insecurity and eventually had to give up his job. He is now settled in a lower position and is much happier than before.

The other comment is with regard to industrial zoning. I recall a factory in South-East Asia which was given permission to be built on a certain site, and the authority must have forgotten about it, because by the time it was built another authority had given permission for a housing estate to be built on an adjacent plot. The housing estate went up and the people who bought homes there didn't know that a factory would be built next to them. This factory, now built, produces a dangerous dust hazard, but there is little that people can do except move out. The factory was put up by permission of one authority and the housing estate by permission of another. This is one of those distressing mistakes that should not have happened: there should have been proper co-ordination between the two authorities.

Bridger: I wonder if Dr El Batawi will accept my growing impatience in listening to him as a compliment, and not the reverse! I wanted to turn the question round. Can he give us evidence of work done by WHO which tells us why the *obvious* isn't done? In writings going back to earliest times—for example, the sayings of Confucius and others—we find a plethora of explicit and implicit exhortations and precepts, but very little attention to finding out why mistakes still happen. We know that they should not, and we even know, not infrequently, what should be done. Why is it that the 'solution' does not happen? This is a much more important question than another list of things that *should* happen. It is the understanding of some of the things that happen, and why they happen, that lies at the root of some of these situations and the hope for the future. Even Professor Phoon's story about the shift leader is, if I may say so, over-simplifying the issue. I have never known a direct cause-and-effect relationship in all the studies I have done. It is not difficult to restructure an organization and bend it in such a way that two good friends can become bitter enemies in a short space of time. As primary patterns of disruption, personality problems as such play far less part than role conflict, socio-technical dissonance, and so on. The importance of Professor Phoon's comments is related to the earlier plea for more money to be deflected from armaments into this area of prevention. We tend, however, not to examine why some of these things don't happen and what the motivation is. Many of these events are controllable, but we must begin to understand the dynamics of the envies and jealousies—and not just the political ones. Why do some economists think of 'economic man', and not the other kind of man as well? Why and how are some of these unreasonable and irrational forces let loose? We cannot find rational solutions to irrational dynamic situations. It is the study of these situations that I would like to see more money going into.

Mars: Harold Bridger's plea, I think, subsumes the query raised earlier: if people *had* known about the problems of the Volta development project before it started, would the same mistakes have been made? His hint is that they would, and it seems very possible that he is right. This approach, I suggest, also throws light on what Professor Phoon has said about problems created by outside specialists who visit for one month and write a book, when there are plenty of local people who already know about a country. I would say that these issues raise questions not just of foreknowledge, the point raised by Lord Ashby, but of what *type* of foreknowledge, which is central to the kind of organizational problems that Mr Bridger was touching upon. We need therefore to examine the irrational pressures that affect not only outside specialists in this respect but local specialists too, and we should look particularly at the organizations from which these specialists operate.

As an illustration, an advertising campaign in the UK some years ago tried to increase the sale of a certain food by associating it with upper-class living: advertisements were put out showing people eating in candlelight, which was supposed to be associated with gracious upper-class living, and the product was prominently displayed. But in the north of England people who eat by candlelight are regarded as having to do so because they have not paid their fuel bills! These specialists, like many others, were remote from attitudes in the local situation.

Let us go back to the example from Zambia that I mentioned earlier (p. 67). The assumptions of people running the health services of Zambia were found by Frankenberg and Leeson[10] to be derived from outside Zambia. They had been trained in industrialized countries and were now part of a world élite. Their idea of medical training and provision was to have a superb teaching hospital. In terms of locally available resources this was disastrous, and it has been estimated that its cost would have provided barefoot doctors for every community in Zambia. This is a question of internal organizational dynamics where the innovators had an externally based reference group.

As another example, Newfoundland when it joined with Canada in 1949 was the poorest province of Canada, and it still is. The Canadian government decided under pressure from the Canadian and Newfoundland political élites to put funds into Newfoundland and raise health and educational standards. But people running the scheme based their ideas on successful innovations *outside* Newfoundland, which meant that funds had to be channelled through democratic councils. Every village that was to get a road was made responsible, through a village council, for allocating people to build the road, and the same with the electricity supply. The only problem was that there were no councils and none could get started! The ethic of these communities was collective self-help on an individual basis and nobody would stand up and take a leadership role. If he did, he would be vulnerable to personal attack. The only people who did any basic organizing were outsiders to the villages: the priest, the travelling merchant, and the school teacher.

Similarly, vaccination and vitamin enrichment programmes couldn't be started because nobody would be first to try it. What happened in overcoming certain vitamin deficiency diseases was that they had to adapt the main manufactured food product to reach these villages, which was tinned milk. By arrangement with the producing company health innovators were able to have the milk enriched with vitamins at the point of manufacture—that is, before it reached Newfoundland.

These examples, besides demonstrating the need for on-the-spot localized studies, also bring us to the bureaucracies that carry out innovation and the fact that one should suspect the role of administrators and specialists within them. By 'suspect', I mean subject their roles to analysis in the context of the organization in which they operate. Most innovatory bureaucracies work on the assumption, for instance, that size is important, so that power in organizations is largely a product of the number of people supervised. It is also often assumed that people learn best by moving upwards from one grade in an organization to another, and that moving upwards essentially involves the control of others. These are doubtful beliefs when one examines how they actually operate. We must also look at the assumptions made by professionals within innovatory organizations. Each profession has its own culture; economists, for instance, are trained to hold certain premises which are often very different from the premises of people at the grass roots as well as being different from the basic premises of other professionals with whom they must cooperate.

Phoon: I didn't want to suggest that every outside expert makes mistakes, and I also do not think that 'inside' experts are infallible. There is no question that everyone should be subject to scrutiny. It is true that some of the 'insiders' are as much divorced from their community as people coming in from outside. It is also true that one often needs someone from outside to look at a situation more objectively. But there are bogus experts, who are experts only by the definition of an expert as a person who is 1000 miles away from home! There is also the point that when someone visits a country, assesses the situation, and thinks up a solution, he feels that that's the end of it. But the problem is still there!

With regard to psychological problems, I am aware that it was not just the shift leader but also the interactions between the people in the shift, but the proof of the pudding is in the eating and when this particular man was given extra training and his confidence was built up, he came back and the sickness-absenteeism rate went down. I know that such conditions are always multi-factorial and complex, and there is always a danger of over-simplification.

Barefoot doctors have been mentioned. Their special advantage is not just the type of training or the type of sociopolitical system; in many South-East Asian countries use was made of medical auxiliaries even before the existence of the barefoot doctors in China who, as we know, are neither barefoot nor doctors. They are selected from their communes and given a short training, and then go back and work in their community. The point that is important and difficult to follow in a democratic society is the selection of these people, which is crucial. In China the man or woman is chosen from the commune on the basis of his or her motivation, whereas in a so-called free or democratic society we advertise in the newspapers, and then select people on the basis of who has the best school-leaving certificates and so on. The medical student is selected on his I.Q. or his educational qualifications or on how he talks during his interview. So a main reason for the success of the barefoot doctor scheme is the motivation of the people selected, who are well known in their commune and recommended by the people in that commune who know their character and motivation very well.

Illich: I want to try to understand clearly the terms being used in the discussion, because I am from a completely different world. The word 'expert': what does it really mean? Does it mean that here is a person who is competent to do something, as midwives are, or does it mean that he is being paid because he has been invested with the role of knowing more than others? Basically, we are constantly dealing with health as if it were a problem for experts, which through the multiplication of experts—whatever the word means—can be improved. In that case, health, or a healthy working situation, is inevitably scarce. The transfer of responsibility for health to experts necessarily renders it a scarce commodity, when these experts are selected by tests, curricula or birth. I just wonder why we don't conceive of the inverse approach to the problem and ask ourselves what are those industrial conditions in which we don't need experts, but where *people* are competent.

Challis: I want to continue that theme, because it also carries on with Mr

Bridger's comments, which I was sad to hear. I feel strongly that in western industry, and particularly in large organized industry, the expert view of systems of control and of management has become so widespread, and also so useful, that we are in danger of driving out the human touch between the various layers in a hierarchy. In fact, in Professor Phoon's example from Singapore, I was heartened to hear that somebody came along and found out that the shift leader was not managing his team; and then somebody else could say to that shift leader 'you are a good man; don't worry'. I'm not surprised that he then went back to work and was successful. He had been given confidence; someone believed in him. It may be a simplified case, but I would like to believe it, and I know instances in my company where this 'simple' approach does work. I have sympathy with Mr Illich's comments because while expert views and external views of a situation are valuable there is a tendency—and perhaps even this symposium displays it—for the expert and the external view to be given more than their due weight. There is also what I call a home view, a tribal view, a 'little people' view, which is a bit of kindliness, a bit of leadership (horrid Victorian word, but it does mean something!) and a lot of encouragement. As industrialization goes to the developing countries it will take with it the rather ruthless, cold, organizational slant. One lesson we are learning in my company is how to come back a little from that clinical stance and become more homely and brotherly. I am anxious that the view from Professor Phoon on the value of simply encouraging a person who feels he is failing, which in a simple way puts him right, is not over-laid by a more clinical view.

Ramalingaswami: I am glad the question of 'experts' has been raised. Although 'expertise' is often equated with competence, in practice it is synonymous with increasing specialization, knowing more and more about less and less, and a certain value system becomes attached to it. A suggestion was made a few years ago that in order to change this value system, one should call the front-line physician—the man dealing with the basic health problems of the community, which is what a particular country requires most—a first-class or class I physician. Then call a man who is working in a district hospital, who is specialized, a second-class or class II physician; and a man who is working in a teaching hospital—say, a neurosurgeon—call him a third-class or class III physician. In other words, the idea seems to be to restore dignity to work that is most relevant to a particular area. I am glad that Ivan Illich asked the question of who *is* an expert.

Bridger: If I were a lawyer, listening to this recommendation for the reversal of the order of status in medical society, I would probably refer to it as 'compounding a felony' or the equivalent of saying that, from tomorrow, we are going to have democracy by order, and it will be *my* order, and not yours! There is a danger that in wanting to remedy certain things we will, without realizing it, be creating another similar problem, but in some other way or in another place.

El Batawi: I want to take up Mr Bridger's challenge. First I should stress that the World Health Organization does not have executive power, nor do any of the UN agencies. Their conventions or recommendations can be adopted overwhelmingly by labour, employers and governments but when everyone goes back to his own country there is very little implementation. Ratification of conventions is a completely different matter from approval in international forums. For example, the representative of a country may come to the World Health Assembly and support the integration of occupational health services but he goes back and does little about it.

A second point is that there are many other constraints besides the financial ones. The total annual WHO budget to care for the health of people throughout the world is about US $120 million, whereas for example the *daily* military assistance to Cambodia was said to amount to US $200 million for a time. So one can understand some of the financial constraints. Other constraints are historical. Public health disciplines evolved as a consequence of pandemics and epidemics. The epidemiological approach was based on communicable disease and an attempt to find and control its sources, for example by sanitation. Physicians were given to understand that public health is limited to sanitation, sewage disposal and water supply, and felt that such work was not as attractive as, for example, curative medicine. So the public health concept had a poor beginning. In the meantime, there was the Industrial Revolution in the 19th century, associated with the exploitation of labour which still exists today; I have found children pulling carts out of small mines and women still employed in arduous tasks in many countries. The Industrial Revolution, through the conscience of society, developed labour-protective legislation which was extended to protect workers against health hazards and accidents at work. This field automatically became the responsibility of governmental labour departments, as it is still in many parts of the world. I have already pointed out how weak this tool is. It is inadequate; its execution is generally poor; and the people who are dealing with it are inadequately trained, particularly in developing countries.

Since then, two things have developed: epidemics and communicable diseases have almost disappeared in industrial countries but more chronic diseases of more complex aetiology have started to appear, and public health practice has begun to emphasize these. But what are public health authorities doing? Almost 70% of the public health effort in many countries is directed towards hospitals and medical care and rehabilitation and very little is directed towards prevention. I have been trying to convince public health planners that workers are a sector of the population who should be cared for. Although this seems obvious, it has not been easy to make people understand the simple fact that workers are affected by the same diseases as the general population, that they are more convenient to reach, and in the framework of public health plans one can have a very effective preventive health programme. Workers' health is still considered by public health planners as the responsibility of employers and labour departments. And, as was said earlier, if in the UK you have so many walls that you are trying to remove in favour of integration of services and you find it difficult, these walls may also exist in developing countries. However, such barriers may be easier to avoid, as the system is in its beginning in these countries.

Ramalingaswami: As Dr El Batawi says, the number of people in the category of the working population is substantial and will increase whether we like it or not. Here is, logistically speaking, a target group—a captive group—where many things we want to do in the community can be done. In India, the organized sector of industries is promoting the family planning movement with considerable success. This success will have a replication effect. The private sector is assisting the Government in employing their trade channels for the delivery of conventional contraceptives to people. Furthermore, we have problems with the evaluation of intervention programmes because of inadequate data, a problem in many developing countries. In the organized sector of industry there is an opportunity of arriving at cost-benefit or cost-effectiveness ratios in terms of the inputs, because reliable data can be obtained and follow-up is possible.

Bridger: I do welcome Dr El Batawi's response to my question, because there is something here that relates more to his *feelings* of where he was than to the cool logic of his paper; I really felt his impatience with society. This is the kind of outlook that I am very glad to see coming out of WHO.

On Mr Challis's points about experts, it is important to add that his company, ICI, has spent more money on the external expertise of behavioural science than any other company, or probably any two or three companies together. But other companies (e.g. Philips) have directed some relevant external social science resources towards the building up of internal expertise, i.e. the development of a variety of 'internal consultant'. One strategy is not necessarily better than another. What matters is the relevance to the particular organization. The problem about the word 'expert' is that we use it for many different purposes. We use it for competence, knowledge and scholarship in certain disciplines or in certain professions. We use it also for people who can be consultative in a certain kind of way—providing help to somebody else, but not necessarily always the 'best' expert in the functional or specialist sense. But how do we provide the kind of experts who can help people to generalize or to provide multidisciplinary working? This would assume an interdependent group situation where members of the work force would need to be committed and be responsible for the group's or institution's objectives.

References

1. INTERNATIONAL LABOUR ORGANIZATION (1974) *Bulletin of Labour Statistics*, special edition, World Population Year
2. EL BATAWI, M. A. (1964) National problems of industrial health. *Journal of the Egyptian Public Health Association 39*, 1
3. WORLD HEALTH ORGANIZATION (1972) Occupational health programmes. *WHO Chronicle 26*, 12
4. EL BATAWI, M. A. & NOWEIR, M. H. (1966) Health problems resulting from prolonged exposure to air pollution in Diesel bus garages. *Industrial Health 4*, 1
5. KOREAN INDUSTRIAL HEALTH ASSOCIATION (1967) *Survey Report on Safety and Health in Industrial Establishments 6*, 4
6. EL BATAWI, M. A. (1969) Respiratory diseases resulting from inhalation of cotton and other vegetable dusts. In *Proceedings of the XVIth International Congress on Occupational Health*, Tokyo, pp. 168-170
7. CHEW, P. K. (1973) Industrial Health Unit, Annaul Report, Singapore
8. OSMAN, YOUSIF (1975) The use of pesticides and protection from their hazards in the Democratic Republic of Sudan. In *Proceedings of the 7th World Congress on the Prevention of Occupational Accidents and Diseases*, Dublin, May 1974, in press
9. EL BATAWI, M. A. (1975) Occupational exposure and control in the production and use of pesticides. In *Proceedings of the IIIrd International Congress on Pesticide Chemistry*, Helsinki, July 1974, in press
10. FRANKENBERG, R. & LEESON, J. (1974) In *Sociology and Development* (de Kadt, E. & Williams, G., eds.), Tavistock Publications, London

The industrialization of medicine

IVAN ILLICH

At this symposium I speak very much as an outsider, as one specializing in the study of mythologies, of gods, who is meeting here people for whom health (or sickness) is an entity that can be operationally verified and has meaning only in so far as it can be verified. If I have to identify myself, I would say I am (with Paul Goodman) a 'conservative neolithic'. I believe that technical progress and changes have considerable impact on possible changes in social structure and on freedom. In more modern ideological terminology, I believe strongly that the material forces of production, when they grow beyond certain thresholds, inevitably have an impact on social relations and structure them in an exploitative way. I therefore feel myself an outsider, because so far in the symposium we have been concerned with more, and better, delivery of medical services, not simply to people who are and might become sick, but also in the form of medical controls over the environment. I believe that there are inherent limits in all industrially organized enterprises, not only in the production of goods but also in the production of services, and that therefore, beyond a certain point, the production of both goods and services results in more unwanted by-products than desirable goods. That is, in any production system that is organized industrially, growing marginal disutilities set in for which, beyond a certain point, as with the Puerto Rican drug addicts of New York, people are willing to pay more even though they know that not only do they get less of a kick, but more damage.

Finally, I am evidently concerned, as a philosopher, with health, but basically in my options I am concerned with what cannot be done under any circumstances without damaging health levels even further; that is, with a proscriptive approach to development, rather than a prescriptive approach which indicates what shall be done. To translate this into the language of Anglo-Saxon legal procedures, there is a concern with the right to adversary procedures for all those who are damaged by industrial growth. I am deeply precedent-oriented, concerned with the juristic reference to what we know about how the human being functions, rather than with that of the educators concerned with utopia. I am also concerned with a participatory approach to health—again, trans-lating this into juristic concepts, with bringing controversy to a board of *peers* rather than experts. I am therefore ultimately concerned with the increased right of people to take care of their health and the health of their neighbours rather than with increased, or more equitable, delivery services which for one or another reason, because of the mode in which they are produced, are scarce. Put another way, I am concerned with how one can stop the increasing trans-formation of social processes into zero-sum games which are a by-product of the progressive institutionalization of values, as opposed to more justly or-ganized zero-sum games.

As a focus on my main theme, I believe that it can by now be observed very clearly that in any major area of the production of a value—of a socially desirable good or service—there are at least two totally opposed modes of production: one which is basically autonomous—for example, the realization of the value of locomotion by walking; and a second, which by definition is heteronomous, which I will call industrial. In this case, something is done *for* me.

To take transport as an illustration of this process, I am picked up in one place, when I cease to be a pedestrian, and I am put down in another place, where again I may become one. The locomotion of human beings is therefore essentially produced in two ways: actively by walking (and bicycles make this mode even easier), and passively by 'transportation'. It can be calculated that beyond a certain level of growth of transportation in relation to autonomous locomotion, certain things will inevitably happen in society. For example, society will spend *more* time on locomotion. In developed countries between 25 and 50% of the total waking time of people is spent in driving cars, sitting in cars, going to traffic courts, going to jail, going to hospitals, driving to the job, and earning the money to pay for the transportation. Forty-two per cent of all the energy used in the US goes into making cars or building roads or operating them.[1]

Second, more compulsory travel is necessary, therefore, which for most people comes in such a way that the typical American spends 1700 hours on his car a year in order to do 7500 miles, which means that per hour of life-time spent on transportation he does about six miles. Whereas 'neolithics' do not walk outside their own house or compound for more than 3% or, if they are nomads, sometimes 4 or 5% of the social time, most people in developed societies are compelled to spend 25% of their time in travelling. And most people have very few choices about where they can go. Therefore acceleration depends on transportation beyond a certain point and means a real transfer of power in the form of life-time from the majority to a minority which profits from it.

The same thing can be said for housing. When it is turned from an activity, as it still is for most people in Mexico, into a commodity, the entire society becomes reorganized so as to make houses *for* people, and as a consequence the law in Mexico now discriminates against houses built to standards which self-building makes possible; such houses are declared insanitary. The sanitary system, the education system, the transport system, the water system are all organized totally in favour of houses built *for* people, the majority of whom are worse off than they were before and are frequently disabled from doing what, from palaeolithic times onwards, they could do.

The same argument can be made for conflict resolution, where metropolitan law and procedure invades and soon submerges and destroys local conflict-resolving mechanisms such as those that still exist in Latin American villages and also operate in India. I live in a village in Mexico where the villagers have decided that health, education and social security will never interfere!

The same can be said about schooling. When a society decides to spend a vast amount on learning, those who have taught themselves will be discriminated against and soon those who have less schooling will find that their being at the bottom of society is compounded with their being drop-outs from school, at one of the sixteen possible levels of dropping-out which constitute the social pyramids of a 'schooled' society.

These developments in transportation, housing and schooling that I have described and this institutionalization of values are identical in rich and poor countries and in socialist, communist or capitalist countries (I leave out China because I cannot speak from experience there). They are therefore resistant to those remedies which are possible within the presupposition in favour of industrially produced 'better' values, as opposed to autonomously produced values. Society is totally reorganized in favour of industrial production.

I am *not* proposing, and it is important that this be underlined, some new kind of irrationalism; in fact, I am asking for a rational analysis (a systems analysis) of the system within which we live. It is not a neo-Luddite approach; I am not trying to suggest that we do away with very high technology, for example the bicycle, which incorporates very real inventions, or, in medicine, the pregnancy test, which is at a tremendously high level of modern technology, or the suction apparatus for abortion. I *am* suggesting that we must come to a new prejudice about the use of high technology, which is now constantly incorporated into systems that are totally in favour of the industrial mode of production, and instead incorporate it wherever we can into systems that are organized for autonomous production. I shall end by explaining why this is so difficult to discuss seriously in most milieus in which I speak, because such a choice cannot be made partially; it can be done only by discontinuing most applications of high technology at the service of centralized or industrial production. It can be done only through voluntary self-abnegation to dreams.

Let me turn to 'health'. I speak here simply as a philosopher who wishes to introduce ideas into the discussion. In no way have I anything to add to the highly expert level of the symposium so far. When I look at man, I see that he is different from the other animals, because he is threatened on three fronts. If he does not succumb to the elements, he will be exploited one way or another by members of his own species. He has to defend himself by techniques and by social and political organization. A third front has always been recognized: man in any society or any culture has to defend himself against and find some way of coping with his bad dreams, which myths traditionally structure and, at the same time, answer. Man is an animal whose survival depends on successful coping on these three fronts, and, if I am right, this is what culture is: one particular form which the viability of the human group can take, in its environment, with its neighbours, and with its particular bad dreams. Traditionally, on the level of bad dreams, only the hero was threatened: he alone wanted to live out his lusty, greedy and aggressive dreams; he broke the taboo. In modern industrialization, by contrast, in my analysis, the effect of having things done *for* us rather than being able to do them ourselves represents a materialization of evil dreams: the transformation of dreams into a ritual activity that goes on within society. I see medicine in these terms. If I understand anything about how the Mexican Aztec descendants among whom I live perceive health, they see it as a coping ability—a way of coping with the environment, with neighbours, and with dreams (in the broadest meaning of dreams), and of coping in an autonomous way with these things.

My strong impression after listening to what has been said so far at this symposium and the general style of the discussion is that medicine is conceived here as an enterprise which maintains people heteronomously in an environment over which they really have no control: not only individual medicine, but also social medicine, which has been mostly under discussion here. It is for this reason that I am somewhat frightened that what we are doing is shifting attention away from interventions with people who are, or might become, sick, towards an engineering intervention in an environment which we know to be of an increasingly sick-making (or pathogenic) nature, and therefore the entire medical enterprise becomes a further 'sick-making' enterprise.

What happens when medicine or health care from an autonomous, culturally and traditionally organized enterprise is turned, not into a modern enterprise through new tools or procedures being incorporated into the cultural prog- ramme, but into one that consists of services which are delivered; that is, into heteronomous maintenance? Beyond a certain point the entire social structure is so rearranged that people increasingly lose their power to do things for themselves. Medicine not only itself becomes, beyond a certain point, a health-denying enterprise on an epidemiologically studied level; it also supports an inevitably 'sick-making' reorganization of all other production sectors, by enabling society to use modern technology in the service of higher productivity and lower total effectiveness.

This statement is difficult to make because of the prejudice with which I began, namely that we want to speak scientifically about health and sickness, and scientific discussion of this matter means that we want our ideas to be capable of operational verification—in other words, measurement. Let me go back to my earlier example of transportation. It is extremely difficult to put into the same model, in order to represent the mobility of individuals within a society, two independent modes of production, namely transportation and locomotion by foot or bicycle. For a variety of reasons the two modes cannot be fitted into the same model. One can speak about the commodity that is being delivered, which in this case is transportation, but it is almost impossible to quantify values that are produced but which by their very nature resist translation into other values, and resist marketing. Walking, for instance, or speaking one's mother tongue, and most of the other things that are beautiful in life, resist precisely in this way transformation from use-values into ex- change-values. For this reason we find a great theoretical difficulty in analysing industrial society (because what I am speaking about is not a contradiction or conflict, but a crisis within an industrial society, where the whole industrial mode of production in all major areas must be limited if we want optimally to increase autonomous production).

In medicine, let us look at what happens in what I call the 'over-medicaliza- tion' of a society, which is what has happened in Mexico where, even though most people still have recourse to the *curandero*, the curandero now redefines himself as *uno doctor*. And the incorporation of the *curandero* into the medical establishment by giving him a certificate, as may also be happening now to the barefoot doctors in China, is in no way an alternative proposal, but it is a more effective, more 'yankee'-like form of industrialization for poor countries.

What happens? First, over-medicalization of a society inevitably produces iatrogenesis (that is, medically induced illness) on three distinct levels. The first area of which we are clearly aware consists of the unwanted clinical side- effects of clinical intervention in people. On a second level, there is the increased creation of 'patients' by the medicalizing of all care, all drugs, soon all prevention, and by finding ourselves as part of what has been aptly called 'patient majorities', so that a man's job itself, as we have been hearing in this symposium, becomes a place in which the doctor has to intervene, or has something to say, if the job is to be kept healthy.

The third level is structural iatrogenesis, which consists in disabling people from even wanting to maintain their own health, which for a human being implies the ability to face suffering. I do not believe that one can speak about human health without speaking at the same time about the ability to cope with pain, with having distinct differences from one another, with impairment, and with the fear of death. I have been making a study of the iconography of the doctor during the past four hundred years. It is extraordinary how recently the idea appeared that it is the doctor's task to 'kill' pain[2]. Pain-killing is a concept that one cannot even translate from American into other languages. The idea that sickness can be eliminated is another of these 'materialized' dreams. The final fantasy is the idea that the doctor can manage not only pain, but also death. In western iconography at least, 'death' appeared as a person for the first time in about 1403. I have collected some 1700 pictures of death represented together *with* the doctor. The first time that the doctor steps between the patient and death is a picture by Klimpt of 1919. Until that time, death teases and mocks the doctor, whenever he tries to interpose himself.

Structural iatrogenesis is, in my opinion, a consequence of the belief that the task of coping with pain, impairment and death can be transferred from the person and his primary group to professional, expert intervention. From being essential experience, with which each must come to terms, pain, sickness and death have been transformed into accidents for which people must seek medical treatment.

What therefore is my concern, with my colleagues, in the seminar that we shall be conducting over the next two years? We are attempting to identify political or social procedures by which people can vindicate their right to the effective use of modern technology (or modern applied science, in other words), for the purpose of their own health. I can illustrate this by an example. I was making the point, at a meeting, that legal situations change in a country because of technological progress. This was in Puerto Rico, where there is a considerable fight going on about abortion. One party is insisting that abortion should be outlawed completely. But once the suction method has come on the market and the pregnancy test has been so extremely simplified, such a law is about as valuable as the laws that are still on the books in New England against masturbation! On the other hand, the other party is insisting that abortion should be strictly reserved to doctors, but paid for by the state. But once the new type of equipment is on the market in a poor society, this is about as intelligent as a law which in the early 18th century in Lima made adultery a crime unless it was committed in a certified and approved bordello. In other words, I am speaking about the de-professionalization of the majority of effective medical curative or preventive technologies and approaches. I think this can be done only if at the same time most of the activities for which doctors alone (or highly competent subprofessionals) can be effective are rendered impossible—in poor countries for economic reasons, and in rich countries for political reasons. There is a major field for research here. It has been shown, for example, that most health interventions that require (apart from hotel services in hospitals) more than a very small investment, say $50, show very quickly decreasing evidence of effectiveness; whereas most of the interventions that are truly effective, if differently packaged and arranged, could probably be applied with many fewer unwanted side-effects if they were used among people who love each other and are concerned, deeply and personally, with each other. So it really becomes a question of de-professionalization, which is more a matter of a legal than a medical approach. In other words, I want to orient our discussion towards the analysis of the hygienic limits to overall industrial growth, and to the industrialization of all major sectors, including the medical sector, rather than towards questioning how man can be increasingly programmed for surviving in a world in which the industrial mode of production exercises an overwhelming monopoly on all forms of value.

Discussion

Ramalingaswami: Your case is clearly not against technology *per se.* Technological developments such as the means of measuring human chorionic gonadotropin in the urine a few days after conception by a simplified technique that can be used by the pregnant woman herself, or a suction apparatus for inducing abortion in the first few weeks of pregnancy, or a live oral cholera or typhoid vaccine—all these are high technology and are needed. The question is one of how man should utilize this high technology to serve man maximally. The present frameworks that we have developed are *not* serving that function. I find myself in considerable sympathy with this point of view. In this connection, it was suggested that physicians are a bottleneck to the spread of family planning, to a replacement of the existing demographic irrationality by a rational policy[3]. There are two reasons for this bottleneck. Firstly, the physicians are not located where they are most needed, especially in developing countries. The majority of doctors are living where the minority of the people are. The second bottleneck derives from the mould in which the doctors have been cast through contemporary educational processes which do not prepare them to delegate functions to others in the health team, to recognize the role of each member of the team, and to act as a leader of the health team. It is, therefore, the manner in which medical personnel are trained and oriented that is one of the basic issues in the translation of new technology to serve human needs maximally. Another point you mentioned interests me—how the relatively simple, local-level mechanisms for resolving conflicts have been replaced by imposed, highly structured hierarchical systems. This is true. We pride ourselves in India on the well-developed legal system we have, by which theoretically everybody has access to justice. In actual practice, if one analyses those who use this judicial machinery, it is a relatively small proportion who go to it, because of the costs involved; or because conflicts among people need to be resolved quickly, else they lose their relevance as conflicts, and the legal process is so prolonged that only those who can afford the cost and time make use of it. One could look at the inadequacy of many of the social institutions that have been built in this way. The question is of how one starts to correct this, since we may not be in a position to start a new system. How does one change? As far as physicians are concerned, I suggest that change must take place in their basic training which should be strictly related to the needs of the society that supports their training at great sacrifice.

White: While Ivan Illich's words are always thought-provoking, I also see a basic contradiction in his philosophy between the statement that he is in favour of a participatory approach in which issues are brought before a board of peers, and not of experts, and his recommendation that autonomy should be put first in every case. Are you for people deciding in large groups what they collectively want, or for each individual satisfying his own needs and only joining small groups for specific purposes when cooperation is necessary? If your answer is that you want people organized in large groups to make decisions, but you want to persuade them in those decisions to subordinate the goal of material comfort to the goal of individual autonomy, they may well ask what the point of autonomy is, if everyone's needs are catered for. When you point to the negative effects that some kinds of material production, of production for comfort, entail—especially those which harm others whether or not they really benefit the user—I am entirely with you. But also there are the material goods which it is feasible for everyone to enjoy, which they want, which you cannot say are in themselves harmful, but which require a social process of production, with division of labour. Could these goods not exist in a good society, an egalitarian society in which issues were collectively decided by boards of peers, even though the production of these goods reduced individual autonomy? Isn't it possible and reasonable to have a flexible division of labour in which each person can do various of the manual, intellectual, and clerical activities to which he is inclined rather than being limited to one job, but unnecessary to insist on individual or small-group autonomy? Autonomy may be necessary to enable ordinary people to escape from a system which forces them to pay for other people's comforts, but when you have achieved a system which does not do this, is there any longer any point in it? And are you any more likely to achieve a state of society in which real autonomy is possible on a mass scale, than a state of society which has abolished the need for it?

Phoon: I am fascinated by Mr Illich's paper, but I am not certain that he has proposed any real solutions. There is no question that we all agree that our society is not as good as it should be, but I am not sure what solutions he is suggesting. He said we should not support enterprises which lead to higher productivity but lower effectiveness—but effectiveness in what sense? He wants higher effectiveness, but higher effectiveness for what?

Secondly, he has said that Americans spend 25% of their time in transportation, but I am not so sure that being confined to 3 or 4 m.p.h. or to foot locomotion is really better than travelling faster! It may be true that we should not travel so fast, but I don't think Ivan Illich has proved the point.

He also discussed over-medicalization, and I am sympathetic to that idea. There is a lot of over-usage of medicines, including antibiotics, by physicians, and I agree with Dr Ramalingaswami that we should reorient medical students in their training and in the delegation of responsibilities. But there must be a balance. Without the advances and intervention of medicine many of us would not be alive today. But is it true, or can it be presumed, that ill-health would lead to more happiness? Mr Illich seems to be advocating the concept of the 'noble savage'. I have seen so many people dying of anaemia, high fever and other illness and I am not sure that they are happier that way. I have seen communities ridden with hookworm infestation and people having children with malaria; their life expectancy is about twenty years. They are not better off that way.

Mr Illich suggested that people want to build their own houses. I certainly don't want to build my house. Are we assuming that manual work is necessarily the fulfilment of man's happiness? In Communist China medical students and doctors are required to do manual work in the factory or in the fields once a year or so, but they are often a nuisance to people on the farms; not being a habitual worker, when you come for one month a year you are not very effective and you do not integrate. Moreover, from what I have been told, there is not much sense of self-fulfilment about this.

He said finally that many medical methods which are cheaper could be more effective than more expensive measures if people loved each other. I agree that we should love each other more, but is there any evidence that this will easily come about? Is this not a thoroughly unrealistic supposition? There is a lot wrong with our society and with the education of health personnel; I am sure we can improve these things. But have we any evidence that societies in the past have been 'better' and have led to more self-fulfilment, and do we have here a hypothesis which is an improvement on this very imperfect model of life that we confront today?

Illich: I am surprised that Professor Phoon believes that medical professional interventions have had anything but marginal effects on the change of disease patterns and that he believes that at present medical intervention has a significant effect on increasing life expectancy, except in childhood, and that he speaks about the effectiveness of doctors as if they were in any significant way necessary to provide the limited number of specific, simple and cheap interventions which effect the enormous majority of 'cures' which scientific advance has made possible. Such optimistic ideologies fit into political rhetoric, but not into this symposium.

This kind of optimism becomes health-denying when it distorts the thinking of a medical planner. This is because on the basis of such optimism an improved level of health means the training of more professionals of different kinds and levels, and the creation of a health care system which turns health into the result of service-consumption. A sober evaluation of the relationship between doctors and health patterns will lead to the contrary policy: namely, the most radical possible de-professionalization of personal and community health care and the largest possible participation of the entire population in health-care activities using the simplest and cheapest devices.

This, of course, is impossible as long as our present unfounded optimism about professional services prevails. It is also impossible as long as we misuse public money for expensive interventions on a few sick people (no matter if they are chosen because they can pay part of the bill, or because they interest the doctors who practise on them) and allow the demonstration-effect of these professional stunts (no matter whether individually effective and beneficient or not) to destroy the basis on which a truly post-industrial system would be built—namely, the belief that scientific progress has carried us beyond the time of the doctor, and that most engineering interventions in people who are or might become sick can be provided by neighbours or members of the community.

I say *most*. I do not want to question that in some few valuable and effective procedures, apprenticeship and experience add to the quality of performance.

But even here I question whether the certification of experts by experts contributes more to the good of the community than selection by satisfied clients.

El Batawi: I share Professor Phoon's feelings here, and it is probably a problem of communication! Physicians and philosophers don't meet very often and they may use a different language. I want to add a point on the question of human adaptability. Throughout time, human beings have adapted to many situations, physical and psychological, and in industrialization, adaptability played an important role. Surely we should exploit this capacity to adapt to the greatest possible extent.

Philip: As a barefoot non-expert, I have become increasingly oppressed by a sense of an air of conservatism in this symposium. It has seemed weighed down by some very unadventurous tacit assumptions. Therefore, I have to say how grateful I am to Mr Illich for putting a cat among the tranquillized pigeons. I had expected this symposium to be operating at a radical level of the type which I have only now found during Ivan Illich's paper. I imagine that he would see my suggestions about low-energy technologies (p. 45) as conformable with what he has in mind.

Porter: I have difficulty in visualizing the nature of the society implied by the philosophy that Ivan Illich has expressed. In particular, thinking about the problems of poor countries, such as the Indian subcontinent, it is conceivable that the sort of society which is implied by his vision is feasible in a country with a slow rate of population growth; but in countries with rapidly growing populations, in order for even a minimum of living standards to be preserved production has to increase rapidly, particularly agricultural production; and while one obviously wants to have low-energy technology, to economize energy, one also wants to economize on capital, and one has to organize that production, and this implies some form of industrial organization. The other point is that even if one likes the 'do it yourself', self-help approach, in very poor countries it is not feasible economically to provide medical services in this way on the level that we have medical services in, say, the UK. It might be useful to explore and define the limits of what people can do for themselves and to determine the stage at which one needs the intervention of professionals. This seems to be a better way of looking at this problem than to go to the extreme of saying that we should not train any more doctors. One needs surely to define the nature of the problems with which doctors and other medical personnel have to deal and to organize the system so that they are used most effectively. A concept that you can do this in an entirely uninstitutionalized way on a self-help basis, in medicine of all things, seems to me to be somewhat utopian.

Jones: I have a sense of *déja vu* here, because I see an analogy with the

Reformation! It was priests then, and it is doctors now; de-professionalization, then and now. Self-help, then and now; spiritual then, medical and environmental now. What Mr Illich seems to imply is that history repeats itself. I don't subscribe to that theory, or to the conspiracy theory of history, but I find your analysis attractive, and I agree; but I would like to be clear about your prescriptions for the future. What are we going to do? Bicycles aren't enough. I don't think de-professionalization in itself is enough.

Illich: I indeed insist on health as a process of adaptation, but a process of adaptation that would result from autonomous—individual or group—coping, as opposed to what results from management or engineering. In this I am a pupil of René Dubos, who said that nothing is more dangerous than man's ability to adapt and now, to *be* adapted, and in his capacity to survive, with increasingly more commodities, on unspeakably low levels of health, on which he is maintained. I want almost to repeat Mr Porter's sentence here, but its inverse; let us explore the limits of what can be done *for* people because, beyond a certain point, if more than that is done for, or given to people, their ability to do the simplest things for themselves must decline, because of the reorganization of the entire society in favour of the 'doer'; and therefore people's effectiveness declines. I pointed out the difficulty in measurement here.

Finally, indeed I am speaking about an analogy to the great invention, the alphabet, which is one of the most admirable technologies, having been invented by the Phoenicians, and printing too, when paper production became possible, that allowed Reformation man to take the pen out of the priest's hand. In a similar way, I am surprised and fascinated by the laws in the US which make it a crime to be found with a syringe in your house.

What can be done? My main concern methodologically is to identify those thresholds (if they exist—and it is my hypothesis that they do) in the power of productive institutions beyond which the institution that does things for people (whether providing goods *or* services) inevitably does things in such quanta and defines things in quanta as minimum requirements, that it imposes an exploitative structure on society. A recent example is schooling; another is the speeding up of people. I am concerned not with what people will do tomorrow but with the conditions that we have to keep away from so that people using high technology, but in a decentralized way, today have more choices for doing different things, with enormously greater effectiveness, than they have ever had before. To take the example of transport: a study has been done which shows that if you develop on our computer model either the greater Paris region, or Mexico, in such a way that nobody can go faster than 20 kilometres per hour, the time spent in transportation could go down from 25% to perhaps double the Neolithic level, perhaps 6% of total time; locomotion would then be increased per hour of lifetime spent from the traditional three kilometres to seven or nine kilometres, which is higher than any standardized locomotion velocity at present anywhere. I am speaking of enormous increases in the *effective* achievement of certain specific social goals, on a level of equity, which are impossible as long as we use certain levels of power.

References

1. ILLICH, I. (1973) *Energy and Equity*, Calder & Boyars, London
2. ILLICH, I. (1974) *Medical Nemesis: The Expropriation of Health*, chapter 6, Calder & Boyars, London
3. POTTS, D. M. (1972) Human fertility in global perspective. *Proceedings of an International Conference on Family Planning*, pp. 1-6, New Delhi [See also Potts, D. M. (1974) in *Human Rights in Health (Ciba Foundation Symposium 23)*, pp. 205-217, Associated Scientific Publishers, Amsterdam]

Socio-environmental consequences
of design

VICTOR PAPANEK

The community of nature—the biotic community which gives mankind its environment—has been upset in a major way already. Many examples of individuals deformed, mentally retarded or crippled by water and air pollution exist. But human generations last too long for us to be able to demonstrate *evolutionary* changes in man—*so far*.

Changes caused by an evolving community can clearly be shown by a certain type of moth. In Helsinki, Stockholm, Copenhagen, Vancouver, East Berlin, Pittsburgh and Manchester, naturalists have collected and studied the peppered moth (*Biston betularia*) for 150 years. This moth has silvery wings with a few dark markings. It lives on lichen-covered trees and is prey to several birds. Beginning with heavy sulphur dioxide pollution about 100 years ago, a new melanic form (mutant) appeared, with wings entirely the brownish-black colour of soot-stained buildings (no silver). Within 50 years the mutant has bred true (in smog-polluted areas) and the original moth has completely disappeared. In Britain it was possible 20 years ago actually to chart areas of heavy pollution by the type of peppered moth collected. Relatively pollution-free areas still yield the original form; the drab melanics breed true in polluted areas. But there is hope: as cities are slowly being cleaned up, the *real* peppered moth has reappeared and the mutant is dying out.

I am *not* saying that people are like moths, but I am attempting to show that this can provide a biological read-out device for the diagnosis of sulphur dioxide pollution.

In one of my books[1] I have suggested that industrial designers, industry and governments should together find out about the social and ecological harm we do to our communities. To blame the mess on a profit-seeking capitalist system is silly: our friends in socialist states have the same problem, as do so-called 'hippies' in 'alternative' communes.

171

To say that technology itself is wrong eliminates the only weapon we have, and would produce a world-wide catastrophe that would be first felt in the Third World.

To opt-out into drug-enhanced communes solves nothing; it is a luxury of bourgeois, romantic youth and, in fact: objective fascism.

Industrial 'growth', if directly exported from fully industrialized countries to those that are still industrializing, has far-reaching social, ecological, ethological and environmental consequences. Some of these consequences are malignant. Their main negative effects are pollution and alienation.

In the 'developed' world we pay for our riches by also living with rising statistics of suicide, vandalism, absenteeism, work-sabotage, 'wild-cat' strikes, alcoholism, violence centred around mass sporting events, crimes against the person, neglect and 'battering' of children, unusually high divorce rates and deviant sexual behaviour, drug use, loss of identity, and, finally, *anomie*.

One way in which I can illustrate how the behavioural sciences can be used in design is with the 'washing-machine in the playground' syndrome. It is useless to build better playgrounds in slum areas where women have no time to supervise their children at play. Instead, we have built a playground in which there is a central, glass-enclosed observation area that is fitted out with washing machines and clothes dryers. Consequently, women can supervise their children at play while doing the wash, and also gossip with one another.

It may be questioned where the 'profit' lies in putting washing machines in playgrounds. May I suggest that 'profit' suffers from bad accounting methods. For example,

   (a) What is 'profit' in a 75¢ copy of the New York *Sunday Times* if the city spends $3 to get rid of each copy?
   (b) Where is the 'profit' in motorways that almost become parking lots on the first day they are open?
   (c) Who pays the taxes that build the roads, that make it 'profitable' to build cars?
   (d) And so on.

We speak about 'pollution through products', but the cycle is more complex than we usually think. It consists minimally of seven parts:

   (a) Natural resources are destroyed; moreover, these are usually resources that are irreplaceable.
   (b) The very destruction of these resources (by strip-mining, open pit mining, etc.) creates a pollution phase.
   (c) The manufacturing process itself creates more pollution (phase 2).

(d) This same manufacturing process also brings about worker alienation and *anomie*.

(e) Packaging (this is essentially a repetition of phases *a* and *b*).

(f) The use of the product creates more pollution and adds 'user alienation' and 'user *anomie*' (phase 3).

(g) Finally, discarding the product creates an even more lasting source of pollution (phase 4).

The intervention of designers must be modest, minimal and sensitive. Thus if we find that the indigo-dying of textiles in West Africa creates major breeding areas for tsetse flies and *Anopheles* mosquitoes, the answer is *not* to get rid of the dying pits, but to introduce biological controls.

If in Lesotho the social life of women is centred around the beating of maize, the answer is not to introduce electric maize-grinding machinery, but to simplify the work and still retain the social grouping.

If it is found that the *Mukwa* (head-band) by which Kikuyu women carry loads in Kenya forms depressions in their skulls over the years, we must examine the entire social context of load-carrying in West Africa before introducing some insane 'improvement', such as motor scooters.

In more fully industrialized countries we can often make the workers' work-life more rewarding and more meaningful to them. I have been involved with companies in some of the Scandinavian countries where it has been found that 'just paying people more money' is never enough. Working with native Scandinavian workers as well as foreign 'guest workers', we found that we could get better job performance and less alienation by abandoning assembly lines and introducing pit-team assembly, complete job rotation, rotating team chairmanship, work hours chosen by the team, extra training in various languages and other skills on company time, and so on. If such work techniques are operated in the most technologically advanced countries in the world, then they must also be built into countries that are not yet fully industrialized. To do otherwise smacks of neo-colonialism and exploitation.

To use another example: more than forty manufacturers all over the world make sewing machines. Each manufacturer has a line of between 5 and 25 different machines. New manufacturers, diversifying into the sewing machine market, then create virtual carbon copies of machines already on the market. What are the facts? The facts are that about 85% of the sewing machines in the world are carried daily on people's heads for a distance of about ten miles. Throughout Africa, Asia, South and Central America and even parts of Southern Europe one can see men carrying foot-treadle-operated sewing machines to the market place early each morning, sitting there sewing all day long, and then carrying the machines back home at night. This is one of the facts that might well result in the design and manufacture of an ultra-lightweight yet rugged sewing machine, hand- or foot-treadle-operated, and easy to repair. The individual profit per machine would be quite low (compared with that on a two-tone Singer-de-Luxe sitting in a fake Jacobean chest of fake rosewood); however, potential sales are likely to be in the range of forty million units initially. With this sewing machine example we have finally arrived at a point of departure. Design then follows the normal pattern of selection and diversification, but using a cross-disciplinary team of economists, anthropologists, *the people who sit in the market place and sew*, engineers, and so on, instead of the marketing department. However, the design process does not stop there. For now we must *prove* our theoretical solution of the sewing machine. This deals with the consequences of our design act, including the political, social, environmental, ecological, ergonomic and economic consequences. What would happen if this sewing machine were in fact to be made? Would it dislocate social groupings in East Africa? Should the machine be made in, say, Nigeria? If it were to be made there, would it help to do the things that design and production in a developing country ought to do?

But before *any* design is done in and for a developing country, at least fifteen questions must be asked. Does the design:

1. Make sense in a country with a labour-intensive economy (rather than a capital-intensive economy)?
2. Make sense in terms of the real needs of a relevant market?
3. Bring about more jobs (without destroying social ties)?
4. Bring about more exports (without tying the country to *kitsch*-making for export)?
5. Bring about new jobs and train new skills?
6. Help the country with its balance of payments deficit?
7. Help to develop intermediate technologies to protect people from cultural loss and ecological imbalances?
8. Help industrial diversification?
9. Stop catering to an élite or a class?
10. Create a national identity for the manufacturing country?
11. Give pride and a sense of achievement to the workers in the developing country?
12. Make it possible for workers to innovate and participate in both the design and the manufacturing processes?
13. Help to preserve non-regeneratable materials and energy sources?
14. Help to bring about decentralized ways of living and working?
15. Undertake to work with low energy inputs?

None of these questions can be answered unless we work as members of a cross-disciplinary team that includes workers and users, since so much needs to be known about so many different fields.

Discussion

Phoon: I have myself been interested in the changes in the car industry in Scandinavia that you mentioned, because I have been involved with car assembly firms in Singapore. I wonder how the team is selected: do the men select their own team, or are they assigned to teams? If they choose their team, what happens if there is a turnover of labour and new recruits come in; to what teams are they assigned? And are the teams allowed to change their members if disharmony arises? Again what happens if there is a laggard—a person who has chosen to be in a team but is found not to be playing his part? Lastly, since this experiment seems to be successful, has it been copied by other car firms, and if not, why not?

Papanek: At the Volvo automobile plant the experiments in 'work enrichment' and 'worker' participation' have now gone on for nearly five years. In the beginning car workers in assembly plants were *put* into teams, with the understanding that they could change to other teams after a few weeks. In this manner a sort of self-selection takes place. Furthermore, assembly teams are designed in such a way that there is complete job rotation within each team. That is, each person does every job. But even getting away from the assembly line and working in a team in which jobs rotate carries along sex differences. It was found, for instance, that component parts of automobiles are too heavy for women to carry easily; it was further found that doing the upholstery carries along the stigma of 'sewing' to guest workers from Turkey, Spain or Greece and is perceived as a 'feminine' skill by them. Hence the size of car parts had to be reduced and the upholstery techniques had to be changed in such a way that they would no longer carry connotations of 'housewifely skills' to men coming from chauvinistic backgrounds. This is part of a continuous process of de-mythologizing the work skills so that it is possible for people to rotate from job to job within the plant. Team leadership rotates as well. The primary allegiance of a Volvo car worker is *not* to Volvo but to his production team. It is the team which by common consent sets work schedules, times and so on.

This also answers the question of what to do with 'laggards'. People unwilling to do their full work are very few because the programme itself places the incentive with the team. Many variations are possible: Turkish workers, for example, enjoy drinking strong coffee while working, hence there are many coffee makers on the work floor of the Turkish team. It is really as simple as that.

I should repeat that Volvo have introduced these various schemes in order to cut down absenteeism, work sabotage, 'Friday and Monday' cars and so on. Some of their more primitive processes have been copied (or should I say adapted) by General Motors, Volkswagen, Fiat and Saab. Companies in other areas such as IBM in its Swedish operation and a toy company in Britain work in a similar way now.

However, having said this, I should add that the energy crisis has intervened in automobile production and all of this has become a rather theoretical discussion point.

Finally, the choice before industry lies between an enormous and therefore costly rejection rate of products or having a work force that is encouraged to experiment and innovate.

Philip: I am interested in Professor Papanek's remarks on the true social and environmental costs of innovations. This is something very important that nobody has yet come to grips with successfully. Of course, the notion goes back a long time. As early as 1912, the Cambridge economist A. C. Pigou set out clearly the discrepancy between the market cost, or the market price of goods, and the social cost[2]. Pigou emphasized that industry need have no concern about the effluents it discharges because any damage done is a social cost and not a private cost; that is, it is not chargeable to industry. He illuminated the difference between *social* and *private* costs through the example of factory smoke, which 'inflicts a heavy uncharged loss on the community in respect of health, of injury to buildings and vegetables, of expenses of washing clothes and cleaning rooms, of expenses for the provision of artificial light, and in many other ways (ref. 2, p. 178).

Conventional cost-benefit analyses, however they are are fiddled, cannot become the desired means of social accounting. There may be some prospect, however, of a mode of *energy accounting*. This would, of course, differ fundamentally from present-day cost-benefit analyses; and I suspect that Professor Papanek has something like this in mind. I believe that this is a matter of great importance, but also of great difficulty. I have worried at this idea for some time, but I confess I am not yet clear how one combines energy accounting of non-renewable energy and of renewable energy, such as solar energy. For all that, it would appear that national planning, or indeed world planning, can only hope to become realistic in terms of environmental issues when we have a more certain way of calculating the social and the long-term costs of what we do. Energy budgeting is a possible way.

Papanek: The true social cost of the things we produce has never yet been calculated. There is room for research here[3]. By combining the skills of economists, social scientists, production specialists and others I feel sure that we could show that the *true* social costs of the things we produce are much higher than a hundred per cent.

Gilson: To go back to some of your inventions which are designed for production and use in developing countries: when you have one of your devices started in a developing country and meeting your fifteen criteria for a successful design, how long in practice do they go on being produced? And how do you cope with a situation where somebody says that this device really needs developing 'properly', and wants to do this, including taking steps which conflict with some of those fifteen criteria?

Papanek: I listed fifteen parameters that deal with the design and production of things in developing countries (see p. 174). *None* of these fifteen questions can be answered unless one works as a member of a cross-disciplinary team, since much needs to be known about many different fields. In practice, nearly all of these devices are 'intermediate' design in nature. They may be used for a year, or three or five years, but no longer than that. Sooner or later local governments will seek to change the device or artifact, since I am then no longer in control, and I can only hope that it will still be responsive to the people's needs.

Dickinson: I am very interested in Dr Papanek's devices, the way they work and the costs he achieves. However, he hasn't mentioned the most crucial problem: although he can design these things, how do we persuade their users to design the next generation of things for themselves? I would like to ask Dr Papanek if he has had any experience of getting indigenous design going, or if he has tried to include, in his designs, 'indigenous' features which would make it easy for local people to adapt them, and enable them to proceed to undertake the next generation of designs by themselves? This point is really a continuation of some of Ivan Illich's ideas. It is in this area of autogeneration and spontaneity that we see the development of any society. The only real development aid that we can give is to help and encourage people to develop their own independent ideas; the only success is when people tell us we are no longer wanted.

Papanek: In getting designs going I have so far always worked with people from the area as part of the design team. This makes it possible for innovation and needs to be voiced from the ground up. The final goal in all of this sort of design occurs when people such as myself are phased out because the people on the ground are able to make their own decisions.

I don't protect my designs because I don't, personally, believe in patents. If people want to to take any of my ideas, they are available freely. If the ideas are complex then I send people information, explaining how to copy them. I feel that ideas should be shared because ideas can be developed much faster than solutions: ideas are cheap.

Naturally, this kind of open system lends itself to abuse. For example, we have developed a very simple tape-player that can be made from locally available materials, and is based on a commercial design which doesn't go into the public domain until a few years from now. The firm in the West could in fact make our model itself and ship it out to the countries for which we designed it. We cannot prevent them, but on the other hand they cannot prevent Nigeria or Tanzania from sabotaging their export by making the tape-players themselves on a village level.

One of the more interesting designs deals with how one could make a better bicycle. Bicycle technology is already far advanced; improvements are hard to come by. However, a young man in Holland has recently designed a so-called 'tin' bicycle. It is better in one important dimension; it can be made by 20 or 30 people anywhere in the world without an extravagant factory process. It makes it possible then for people anywhere to get the technology and begin using it to make bicycles for themselves and their neighbours. And in this they cannot be outdone by any large corporation; in fact they will be able to vary the basic design to fit their varying needs.

Mars: What you seem to have done, Professor Papanek, in your approach to innovation, is to have made a very good marriage of local technology and local needs. It is often the problem, in all sorts of development, that there isn't this kind of marriage between the innovators and the 'innovated with'. But how do you go about finding out what the needs are? It is relatively easy then to discover the local technological basis, but I am interested in the problem of discovering the needs.

Papanek: I can only say that we do this with great difficulty! It takes a very long time to discover the needs, and this is usually established by the people there. To me, the hardest job is to find a way in which I can make my professional skills as a designer totally available to the local people, who at this point don't understand the 'manipulative magic' of what it is that I do.

References

1. PAPANEK, V. (1971) *Design for the Real World: Human Ecology and Social Change*, Pantheon Books, New York
2. PIGOU, A. C. (1912) *Wealth and Welfare*, Macmillan, London
3. PAPANEK, V. (1975) *How Things Don't Work: Learning to Cope with Technological Change*, Pantheon Books, New York

Environmental and social problems arising from industrial growth

E. J. CHALLIS

The growth of industry produces wealth and raises the standard of living in the industrial communities. However, the economics of big-scale operation soon force the construction of large industrial plants which replace the former small units. Problems of size, of complexity, of operation and of pollution follow in the wake of these changes and the results can be seen in every industrialized nation in the world today. The general pattern of industry is followed by the chemical industry, but some of the problems become intensified by the nature of chemical production, which lends itself readily to automation. Automatic control and operation give a strong impetus to the favourable economics of big-scale operation, and also facilitate the manipulation of high-energy reactions in arduous conditions of temperature and pressure. Thus modern chemical industry tends to be capital-intensive, employing relatively small numbers of people. The plant units are massive in size, and are often grouped together to form a major factory; in this way the chemical products from one operation can be cheaply transferred to another for further processing. Finally, the nature of the chemicals in the production processes often present greater potential hazards to people and to ecology than the simpler materials processed in engineering or other large-scale industry.

The problems of industrial growth in relation to the community surrounding any factory fall into two classes. Firstly there are the problems of pollution, as observed by the degree of disturbance to ecology within the local area. Secondly there are the problems of the social impact which large industrial factories make on the surrounding urban communities.

PROBLEMS OF POLLUTION

These arise mainly in the air, the water, and to an increasing amount as

179

nuisance from noise. All three problem areas are intensified by the large scale of operation adopted by modern industry. It is worth remembering that a polluting effect is only observed when the local ecology becomes disturbed or shows signs of overstrain. Thus, small emissions of dust or of sulphur dioxide gas can be dispersed easily and will rarely give rise to a polluting effect. The sewage from a small village can be discharged into the local river with minimum treatment and will give rise to no pollution of the aquatic regime. The massive discharge from a large city, or the discharge of effluent from a large factory, can overwhelm the natural purifying powers of the same river and gross pollution will result.

This simple statement on the nature of pollution is necessary because it demonstrates two points. Firstly, there is a considerable natural purifying power in the environment which it is right to use in abating the effects of any effluent. Secondly, the pollution arising from large-scale communities of people is similar to, and just as much a problem as, the pollution arising from large-scale factories. These points are often overlooked when pollution control is being discussed. There is no need to demand the 'nil pollution factory', there is equally no need to endeavour to make the 'nil pollution community'. When discussion rages about the principle of 'the polluter pays' it is often not realized that it is as costly for the community to make its contribution towards progress as it is for the industry which brings wealth and a high standard of living to everyone in the surrounding community.

In this short paper I do not intend to say much about the technology of pollution problems, or the technology of their solution. In general, there are very few pollution problems for which technical solutions do not already exist. The rate at which the means of abating a pollutant are applied is controlled mainly by the cost of the measures to be taken, the disruptive effect on industrial and community life of too rapid a change, and the existence in the whole community of a general will to pay for the abatement methods.

A few general examples will demonstrate the truth of this statement. Sulphur dioxide is a toxic gas which is present wherever coal or oil is burnt. There are many examples of industrial communities that have suffered gross polluting effects because the concentration of sulphur dioxide has been high in the local air. The local solution is now well proven in practice and relies upon dispersion or suppression. But high chimneys cost more money, and industry is reluctant to spend the extra. Equally, the use of alternative low-sulphur fuels by the community is expensive and people are reluctant to buy them. In England, the success of the Alkali Inspectorate in promoting and enforcing a high-stack policy for industry has been matched by the success of the Local Authorities in establishing clean air zones in housing areas. Yet both policies had a very

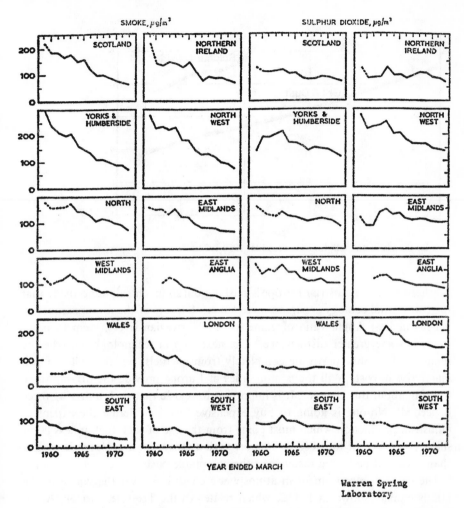

FIG. 1. Trends in urban concentrations of smoke and sulphur dioxide in various regions of the UK (data from Warren Spring Laboratory).

slow start, and have gathered momentum only as the general will towards achieving a cleaner atmosphere became stronger.

Fig. 1 shows the overall effect of these two policies on the air over England today. Clearly there have been big improvements, even though the total tonnage of fuels burnt has risen. In many areas the improvement has satisfied the local people, but is this a permanent solution? Industrial areas become more concentrated, chimney stacks become higher, and there are some fears that the

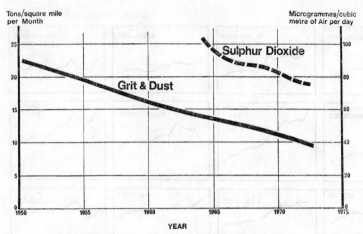

FIG. 2. Trends in air pollution on Teesside, 1950-1973.

northern part of industrial Europe is pushing out so much sulphur dioxide that the continental ecology is beginning to suffer. Surveys of the disappearance of lichens in East Anglia, and of game fish in Norwegian rivers, seem to point towards some greater disturbance. The next step in technology must be the removal of sulphur partly or completely from all fuels, but this will cause a major rise in cost. Will the communities of Europe provide the driving force to bring about this change? It is important to realize that such a driving force is needed. No-one is going to buy expensive fuel, or tolerate the expensive industrial production which must come from the use of such fuel, unless he or she is convinced of the need to support such a move. In a democratic society change cannot be forced faster than the acceptable pace.

The general improvement in atmospheric conditions over the whole of the UK is equally shown in Fig. 2, which relates to the Teesside area of North-East England. The area contains large concentrations of heavy industrial plant, mainly for steel and heavy chemical production. One of the contributions to the improvement has been the quite dramatic fall in the emission of sulphur dioxide from a large chemical factory in the last few years. Fig. 3 shows this change, which was the result of completing a planned closure of several major plants and replacing other plants by modern process units. The rate of improvement was clearly visible as an elimination of smog formation in the industrial area around the factory.

Atmospheric conditions had been quite unacceptable to the local community for a number of years before this change. A big change could have been made sooner, but the closure of plants would have thrown people out of work and

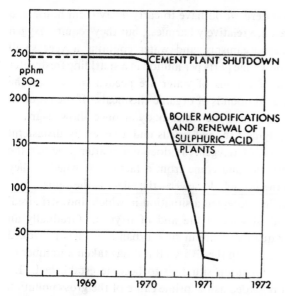

FIG. 3. Changes in atmospheric sulphur dioxide concentration (parts per hundred million, maximum 3-minute mean) around ICI Ltd, Billingham.

seriously reduced the earning power of the whole industrial complex. Such a change would not have been to the overall benefit of the community or the industry. The 'best practicable means' philosophy used by the Alkali Inspectorate, and now incorporated in the control philosophy of other regulatory authorities, avoided a discontinuity in the economic life of both industry and the people in the area. Progress was made, but at a rate which could be afforded.

Problems of air pollution are mainly due to the emission of sulphur dioxide or dust. In earlier times there was also a problem from smoke, both industrial and domestic. The high price of energy has helped to eliminate smoke problems in industrial communities. Householder and factory manager both realize the waste of money which is signalled by a cloud of smoke coming from a chimney, and the skies above industrial nations have rapidly become cleared of this pollutant as energy costs have risen. Certainly there is no justification, either technical or economic, for the continued production of black smoke.

Problems of water pollution are more difficult to tackle, and have come into great prominence partly as the result of the increasing size of urban groups, and partly as the result of the widespread use of chemical products in industry and in the home.

Liquid effluent problems arise from the multitude of organic chemicals which the drainage systems of the modern world have to carry away from house and factory. Often these chemicals are relatively harmless, but they require oxygen for their degradation by microorganisms, and water contains a very small amount of oxygen—perhaps only nine parts per million in a sparkling freshwater stream. Thus many millions of gallons of water are needed to provide the oxygen to clean up a few hundred pounds of organic chemicals. If the required amount of oxygen is not present then the water body at once shows signs of gross pollution. Black mud, dying fish, evil smells and a generally distasteful appearance all result from lack of oxygen. It does not matter whether the offending chemicals are 'synthetic' and come from a factory or whether they are 'natural' and come from the household sewer—the effect is the same.

For many decades, the UK has accepted a situation in which 'industrialized' rivers were often totally dead, devoid of life and of oxygen. Gradually an increasing desire for a better quality of life in such urban areas has provoked demands for a programme to clean up the rivers. But it has taken a number of years for the full facts of the pollution situation to become established. Industrial pollution was at first regarded as the prime cause of the gross pollution which could be seen. Only later has it been realized that the size and concentration of urban areas gives a problem of sewage which often matches, and sometimes surpasses, the pollution coming from the industrial factories in these same areas.

Sewage treatment is now well understood technically, but is still an expensive operation. Treatment of industrial liquids is even more expensive and the technical problems of finding a treatment process with acceptable costs are very much greater. Technical solutions exist today for all the liquid pollution problems in industry, but the application of some of the methods of purification would make an industrial operation prohibitively expensive. A compromise has to be found between acceptable standards of purification and acceptable cost burdens.

The problems of pollution by liquid effluents are particularly severe in the chemical industry. Many chemicals that can be degraded quite easily in very dilute sewage liquids are difficult to handle in the stronger streams leaving a chemical plant. Complex chemical treatment methods are often expensive to install and run and for a small factory it will be better to put the effluent into the town's sewage. Good dilution will enable ordinary sewage treatment to apply and the factory can pay the community for the cost of treatment. Very large factories have big effluent flows and such a solution is not possible.

An example of the interdependence of industry and the community in the area of liquid pollution control is demonstrated in the North-East of England on the River Tees. The Teesside conurbation of about 450 000 people has been dominated by massive industry, both steel and chemicals, for half a century. During that time the River Tees has been degraded by industrial and urban pollution to such an extent that the twenty miles of industrial reach of the estuary are classed as 'grossly polluted'. In fact in the late 1960's it was shown that the Tees in this mid-industrial reach became anaerobic in the summer and putrefaction set in, with the production of methane from the river mud. This situation was disturbing to a few people in Teesside, but neither the community nor industry made major steps to clean up the situation until 1969. At that time a joint committee representing industry, the community and the River Authority was set up to plan a stage-by-stage improvement in the situation. The declared aim was to make the Tees suitable for migratory fish at all states of the tide and freshwater flow. The target date was 1980. Initially it was thought that very large sums would have to be spent by the community and by industry. A great deal of the pollution load came from massive ICI chemical factories on the north and south banks of the Tees, and early estimates of the cost of abating the pollution from these factories indicated that some £20–30 million would be needed. Similarly, a consultant firm engaged by the community showed that there would be an enormous amount of civil engineering work in re-sewering the area and providing several major sewage treatment plants. Capital works of about £30 million were envisaged.

The joint committee appointed a technical Working Party to examine the whole problem and make a plan of stagewise improvement which would minimize the cost and spread the impact of the capital spending. A great deal of technical information was gathered and the special expertise in ICI was freely given to establish the environmental and biological facts about the pollution of the river. A mathematical model of the pollution pattern and the hydraulic pattern in the twenty miles of industrialized river was created. This joint study proved very beneficial. Use of the model showed that a much cheaper sewage scheme for the community would have almost the same beneficial effect on the river as the original very expensive scheme. It also became clear that industrial pollution further up the river needed to be considerably reduced, whereas that entering the river near the sea could be reduced to a lesser extent by making use of the natural purifying power of the fully oxygenated seaward end of the estuary. The study also set targets for industry, and within the two great chemical works these targets were used to set in train a series of stagewise improvements in effluent purification.

As a result of this programme, improvements in the River Tees have been made without a massive dislocation of industry and with the minimum expenditure of public money in the community. The programme has nearly reached the end of Stage I, due in 1975. Fig. 4 shows the deterioration that

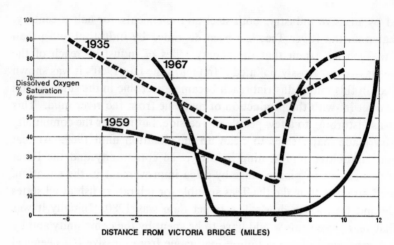

FIG. 4. The distribution of dissolved oxygen in the Tees Estuary in 1935, 1959 and 1967.

has taken place in the last 30 years, in terms of dissolved oxygen. Major improvements in the oxygenation of the river have been demonstrated over the last few years. Biological studies, made by ICI and by some northern universities, have also established an improvement in both flora and fauna.

Within the big chemical sites the setting of time-based, staged improvement targets has enabled a great deal of abatement work to be done without the massive expenditure which it was originally feared would be required. Fig. 5 shows the reduction achieved on the Wilton Site during three years of the campaign, the measure of pollution used being the 'biological oxygen demand' (BOD) of the effluent stream. It was originally thought that such a reduction could cost about £10 million. In fact the progress has been made by detailed studies, by advances in research on particular effluent streams, and by the installation of small, specialized treatment plants in various parts of the Works. So far this work has cost around £3 million.

Two general lessons can be drawn from this successful attack on a major effluent problem: firstly, the value of obtaining good scientific facts about a polluted river before starting on a clean-up programme, and secondly the value of close cooperation between the community officials, the River Authority and industrial experts. The Tees Estuary has truly been treated as a 'systems study', with benefit to all the contributing parties.

There is however, a social problem in such cooperative efforts. This arises from the establishing of mutual trust between the various Authorities, the public and the industry. While it was not difficult to establish the right attitudes in the

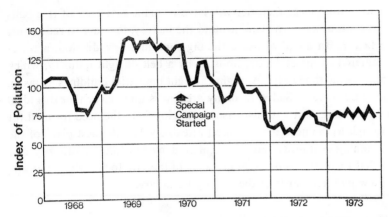

FIG. 5. The improvement in effluent from a large chemical factory, the Wilton site of ICI Ltd. The index of pollution is the 'biological oxygen demand' (BOD). Production doubled in the time interval shown.

official committees where technical men talked together and had mutual respect, it was much more difficult to convince the public and their elected representatives that the scheme of phased 'clean-up' was the right one. There was suspicion that industry was dragging its feet and unduly influencing the study to the detriment of the community. A considerable amount of senior executive time was put in by industry and by officials of the Local Authority in meeting groups of people from the community and explaining what was going on. Joint meetings, in which the platform was shared by industry, the Local Authority and the River Authority, were also held. The outcome has been a step forward in public participation, but has not been easy. This point is mentioned as having some relevance for other areas in Europe and elsewhere, where a massive pollution problem either exists or is likely to arise.

Finally, I would like to mention the growing problem of industrial noise. The problem is not that of protecting workers against the effect of noise inside the plant but of reducing the annoyance to a community outside the factory gates that is produced by a comparatively low level of industrial noise. The problem is much more acute where factories are in continuous operation. Once again, the increase in size and scale of industry and the higher capital intensity of such operations increases the driving force towards 'round the clock' working. A large industrial complex may be using several hundred thousand horsepower in its plants and the resulting hum may not be a disturbance during the day, but may cause bitter complaint if it goes on beyond midnight. The problem is intensified in heavily industrialized areas where land is at a premium and housing gets closer and closer to the main factory areas.

It is likely that future large factories will have to make more use of tree belts and artificial contouring of the land around the factory, in order to reduce the annoyance factor. In an ideal world the big continuous-production factories would be buffered from residential housing by a belt of light industry, which works during the daytime only. At night the light industrial buildings act as an effective acoustic screen. Sadly, in many areas it is quite clear that this ideal has not been realized. For various reasons, ranging from the need for land for housing through to the need for increased rateable value, the best plans of the Regional Planning Authority have been altered by the Local Authority and spoiled, so that there are many large factories in the UK today where housing is within a few hundred yards of the factory boundary.

PROBLEMS OF SOCIAL IMPACT

Growth of industry brings social problems not related to the conventional factors of pollution. Big-scale operation is economic, but its size tends to submerge the identity of the individual. As a result individual workers in a large factory feel at the mercy of a faceless system and this produces a general feeling of resentment. The same reaction can occur in the community where massive Local Authority establishments can become quite dominant in community affairs. A further problem lies in the physical size and extent of modern large industrial plant. Unless care is taken in the layout of the plant the individual feels overwhelmed by a labyrinth of narrow plant roads, high buildings shutting out light, and a general effect of domination by massive plant and equipment.

All these points tend to produce a dissatisfaction with industrial life which overshadows the very real benefits that industrial wealth has brought to both the individual working in the factory and the community surrounding it.

These problems are very much of the 20th century and can be solved if they are tackled vigorously. It is no solution to put back the clock and return to 'cottage industry'. The higher standard of living which everyone in an industrialized nation enjoys will not be given up by most people without a struggle. Indeed the choice is not a real one, because it is possible to solve the social problems of bigness by pro-active methods, rather than by looking wistfully at the past.

To illustrate some of these points I shall refer to the growth of the chemical industry in the conurbation of Teesside. In the 1930's the Tees conurbation was suffering marked industrial depression resulting from the closure of small steel and engineering Works and the general depressed business conditions. A synthetic ammonia factory was started at Billingham on the north bank of

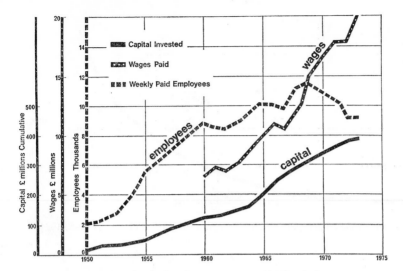

FIG. 6. The growth of the Wilton Works of ICI Ltd, 1950-1973.

the Tees and was rapidly expanded in the next two decades to form a large complex of plants making heavy industrial chemicals and fertilizers, and the beginnings of a petrochemical production. In the 1950's a new complex was started at Wilton south of the Tees, and in the next 25 years it also rapidly expanded to become the largest chemical complex in Western Europe with its production based entirely on petrochemicals.

The growth of both these complexes has undoubtedly brought great wealth into the area. Fig. 6 shows the growth of the Wilton factory over the period 1950–1973. The wages paid represent a very large introduction of wealth into an area where the total working population engaged in industrial operations is around 50 000 out of the 450 000 people living in the conurbation. Fig. 7 shows the rise in the amount of rates (local taxes) paid by ICI. This money represents 'disposable income' for the Local Authority and can be put to use to provide swimming baths, town centres, conference halls and other capital items which increase the public standard of living.

This rise in wealth has had a strong social impact on the area, not all of it favourable. In the 1930's ICI recognized its domination in the area and adopted a paternalistic approach to its work force and to the neighbouring communities. Company housing was built; the standard was in advance of its time and still represents reasonable housing forty years later. A Company Club was built and became the focus of social life in a large area. It was undoubtedly the best-quality Club for miles around. Company staff and payroll were encouraged to

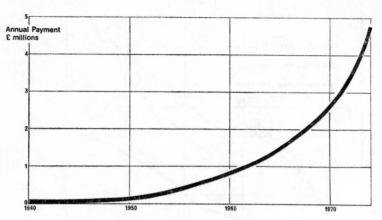

FIG. 7. The rise in the annual rates (local taxes) paid by ICI Ltd (Teesside), 1940-1974.

take office in the Local Authorities and a great deal of voluntary work was done and voluntary provision of money was made. This was very welcome to the community in the 1930's, but by the 1960's the higher standard of living that had been achieved in the area, coupled with the change in social climate in the whole of the UK, caused a resentment of the Company's domination. The new Wilton complex in the 1950's did not provide Company housing but did provide a Company Club. Ten years later that club and its amenities had been overtaken in standard by half a dozen such facilities in the Teesside community and its influence as a centre for the work force had become relatively insignificant.

It was necessary to react to the changed social climate by withdrawing from a paternalistic attitude with the least fuss possible. Company housing was handed over to Local Authorities and the many informal and voluntary social operations were either regularized or handed over to the new Social Services Departments in the Local Authority. At the same time it became necessary to spell out for the very first time in public how much, in terms of wages and rates, the Company benefited the community. This became necessary because of the emotional problems engendered in the community by the obvious change in the Company's role. In the 1970's the situation has become more stable, with Local Authorities spending large capital sums on community facilities, and the Company restricting its position to the formal release of people for Local Authority service and a slowly increasing amount of informal voluntary participation in public services, for instance in youth service adventure training.

The social problem of size in terms of domination in the community has not been solved, but the social upheavals of the 1950's and 1960's have largely abated. A new role for the chemical company has been found and it is interesting to notice that the British Steel Corporation, the other major employer in the area, is beginning to come to a similar stance.

Problems of social engineering within the factory units still remain. Considerable advances were made in factory design and layout in the period between the construction of the Billingham complex in 1930–1940 and the Wilton complex, which was largely built during 1950–1970. They include the setting back of building lines at Wilton to reduce the dominating effect of large buildings and equipment, the laying out of green lawns which are kept properly maintained and mown, and the use of flowers and shrubs in grouped beds at key places in the factory layout. It is clear that Wilton is a 'better place to work' in general than Billingham, and efforts are now being made to update the layout of the Billingham factory.

The 'facelessness of the bosses' in a modern large organization is a problem still to be tackled and solved. The effective use of management systems in the 1950's and 1960's has improved organization and control, but has tended to reduce the emphasis on personal contact as a way of getting things done. In the last few years there have been major efforts within ICI to bring back into prominence the person-to-person link at all levels in the factory. There are some signs that this endeavour is improving the general human climate in which the large numbers of people in the organization work day-by-day. The problem is very much one of size and is best tackled by breaking up an organization of 10 000 people into small identifiable units which associate with a natural work group and a natural work place.

LESSONS FOR THE FUTURE

Looking back over the past decade one can see major advances in the handling of the big industrial problems that arise both from pollution and from the social impact of large industry. What lessons can be learned from this experience that will be helpful in the future? I believe that some general points emerge that will help to correct problem areas in existing large industrial communities and also can be applied to forestall such problems arising in new industrial developments, particularly where these are to be sited in traditionally non-industrial communities.

On matters of pollution, it cannot be stressed too much that size is a major factor. A small factory can emit amounts of pollutants that will become quite unacceptable as the factory size increases. This arises from the fact that the environment has a tolerance of most pollutants and can absorb a certain concentration of industrial emissions without a polluting effect arising. Due regard should be paid to the ability of the environment to carry out this function. However, emissions which go beyond that limit will cause pollution and must be controlled.

Emission-control equipment is most cheaply built into a factory at a time when new capital investment is being made. It is nearly always more expensive to modify plant and equipment after they have been installed in order to achieve some better standard of emission.

In looking at any given situation where industrial operation is making, or will make, an impact on the community, we must reach agreement on standards of control for emissions, and these standards should be seen against a background of expected industrial growth. Consultation between regulatory officials, factory managements, and community leaders is a valuable way of making progress, either in setting standards for a new complex or in improving standards in an existing situation. Such consultation should be guided by three principles.

Firstly, stagewise improvement should be planned over a period of time into the future. This is helpful to industrialists who can plan their technical operations. It also helps the various regulatory authorities involved, who will be able to monitor progress against fixed targets. Such a plan is also valuable to the community, which is protected from the industrial disruption caused by the sudden application of a high standard of effluent control but which is also given a feeling that progress can be seen to be made year by year and that 'something is being done'.

Secondly, experience has shown that most pollution problems are less expensive to solve than appears at first sight. There is considerable value in applying classical scientific research methods to problems of this type: first establish the facts, then break the problem into component pieces, then set out a programme of action.

Thirdly, the principle of human involvement is very applicable both in the technical area of pollution control and in the social engineering area of community impact. A Works Manager who really believes that he must try to reduce emissions from his factory can work wonders by walking round the plant and tightening up on a hundred small emissions. This will ease matters long before the technical design team have produced their major scheme for effluent abatement, and it will certainly reduce the cost of that scheme. In a similar fashion, the involvement of community leaders and groups of people in the community who are not employed industrially can go a long way to solving some of the problems of industrial impact. Simple devices such as Works visits by members of the public, talks by managers to community groups, and the use by the community of industrial talent and industrial facilities for public works, all help to increase the understanding between the community and the industrial firm.

These principles apply to all situations whether controlled by private enterprise or by the State. However, where State control is absolute and the industrial organizations are run under State ownership, it is still very important to make the distinction between the management of the industry, the State Regulatory Authority and the community leadership. These three groups interact and must be seen to play their part in reducing the impact of industrial growth on the community outside the factory.

Discussion

Dickinson: You mentioned that in the improved factory layout of the Wilton Works you have included flower beds and lawns. Do you tell the workers that they are, in fact, partly to improve the appearance of the works and partly as indicators of pollution?

Challis: No. We don't *say* anything about them. These are intelligent people and they know that roses curl up and turn brown at the edges if you dose them with sulphuric acid vapour. We don't say anything, but somebody will occasionally say 'I think the factory site entrance looks a mess; can't we have some rose beds there?' and if that is said, we say yes.

Dickinson: Would there be any advantage in actually saying that you are selecting plants which are indicative of certain types of pollution, as generalized, public monitors which everybody can see?

Challis: I attack it the other way round. In a big factory like this, one square mile in area with 10 000 people working in it, participation by the workforce, and the public, is a key thing. When ordinary people come in from the neighbourhood I may point out the flowers and make a joke about them not being plastic. But I don't stress the fact that the existence of flowering plants indicates a low level of pollution. In technically based industry there is a tendency to crush people with a heavy supply of information. The key point is to underplay the technology and give ordinary folk a feeling of confidence. Just let them come into the factory, feel the grass and breathe the air.

Bridger: How much participation is there in the development of these ideas, as distinct from thinking them out *for* people? I am bearing Ivan Illich's paper in mind.

Challis: In the original concept of the factory there was virtually none. The idea of opening up the layout, having flower beds and so on was a purely executive concept. In the last ten years ICI have bought a lot of consultancy, and some of it has stuck, on the subject of how you get a workforce of 10 000 feeling that it is part of an organic entity. The overall application of consultants' theories of management is the use of informal conversations. We have shop level informal conversations, where people *do* talk about the grass looking a bit long or the fact that construction traffic has been running across *their* lawn; and once people are talking like that, you are beginning to get somewhere. People who talk like that have identified themselves with belonging to the Works as a whole, and it is then easier to make progress in participation at all levels.

Jones: There is a difference between participation and consultation, which is what you seem to have been going for. Participation is when one contributes to joint executive decisions; consultation is when one listens to other people, but then makes one's own decisions. Where is the balance, between the management and the employees' contribution?

Challis: The balance, which of course is never struck formally, is about 15–20% genuine participation; the rest is consultation. But participation is somebody saying that construction has driven over 'our' lawn; it may be a small example, but it is there. Consultation is much more talking about the layout of new plant, where we ask for views and we take them into account.

Jones: I would not call that participation. One could say that at that low level it is essentially a public relations exercise.

Challis: Many people in Teesside are very cynical about what the company tries to do. This is something one has to ride. My colleagues get upset when we divulge some information in the local press and people say that we have only done this because we need a good image in order to facilitate the acceptance of our industrial plans. Nevertheless, in an industrial situation which historically has moved from paternalism through to attempts to get participation, you have to do experiments. A cynical view will be taken, but ultimately the proof of success is whether there is a better feeling inside the factory. That feeling is almost *animal*, but it is real; and we have a better feeling than ten years ago. You can say cynically that ten years ago it was very poor!

Jones: Do your employees' attitudes reflect attitudes in the community?

Challis: In our recent endeavours we have tried to involve the community by bringing them in, talking, and letting them walk around and make their own value judgements, rather than give press hand-outs, talks and so on. Bringing ordinary members of the public into a factory is a key thing. These visits are not highly formal Works visits with a great accent on technology. They are visits carefully arranged to ensure that ordinary work people are responsible for taking their neighbours round; this cuts the Works down to size, and makes high technology into something which is reasonable to understand. It also helps the man to identify with his own plant and be proud of it, and you can see this happening as he shows his neighbours round.

Holland: In this symposium I have been struck by the lack of hard evidence available on the subject of pollution, and by the absence of ambitions towards evaluation. It is surely crucial, in all the work being done, to try to understand what effect, if any, a change in the environment produces. One of the lessons learnt on Teesside seems to be that it is necessary to undertake appropriate cost-benefit or cost-effectiveness analyses. The annual reports of the Medical Officer of Health for Teesside show that the infant mortality rate in Cleveland has changed over time. Infant mortality is much higher in areas of bad housing than where rehousing has taken place. Of course there may be some selection in the families that have been rehoused, but this still seems to indicate that improvements in environmental conditions have been associated with some measurable impact on well-being.

If only housing policy-makers in Cleveland and elsewhere had been courageous enough to do a proper controlled experiment in rehousing, we might now have a better idea about whether the measures taken were really beneficial to health and welfare. And this raises an important general point. In science, we undertake investigations according to rigorous criteria in order to assess the effect of a change in a particular process or experiment. In government policy-making, or in any social policy change, we tend to rely on assumptions and are rarely willing to be exposed to strict experimental evaluation. Such evaluations would be relatively easy to set up when any new measure is introduced since it is unlikely that everyone could be offered the new facilities immediately. If we followed the procedure of random allocation of new housing, for example, it should provide the policy-maker with a clear evaluation of the effect of different options and with useful information for future planning.

El Batawi: In order to evaluate a health programme one needs certain criteria and parameters to measure: for example, the prevalence of a disease before and after an intervention is necessary for us to evaluate its effectiveness. With respect to cost and benefit, this is one of the difficult things to assess because the benefit is 'health' and in most cases it cannot be quantified in terms of money. In occupational medicine we may say that the lowering of absenteeism or of payment of compensation, and lower costs for medical care and hospital treatment, can be a quantitative measure of effectiveness. As an example, an attempt is being made in the USA in a steel industry to introduce preventive health measures. The factory was hazardous in many ways: it had dust and heat hazards, for example. A decision was made to make certain interventions. The parameters measured beforehand were the rates of sickness, injuries, accidents and absenteeism. The experiment will last about five years, so that the returns after changes have been introduced can be seen.

Secondly, in connexion with Mr Challis's remarks about developing a large industry and providing facilities, improving the area visually and making people happier, these things can be found in developing countries, sometimes to people's surprise. In Taiwan, Dr Sakabe and I visited a glass factory which is connected with the Pittsburgh plate-glass industry. It is air-conditioned; it employs about 5000 people. They have comprehensive health care programmes and complete control of hazardous exposures at work. There is no pollution, and there are flowers all over the gardens; although the factory also contained many potential hazards, they were brought fully under control. Such examples do exist in developing countries, and they act as demonstrations to other employers. Another scheme that Dr Sakabe and I were planning to implement, to educate employers, was to show them what would be the benefits of introducing measures of environmental control and preventive health services in terms of the increased output of the factory. However, this plan was unfortunately discontinued because of changes in that country.

Gilson: Something lacking in this symposium so far is a call for quantitative evidence of the beneficial and evil effects of industrialization in developing countries. It is a common failing that when such industrial projects are started, much money goes into the project itself but none is set aside for assessing what is happening. Unless this assessment is made a separate enterprise, it tends to get lost in the whole project. The result is that the net effect will never be adequately documented, and progress to the next stage will be impaired by lack of quantitative information about past success and failure. For example, the UK Government has been spending money on advertising to counteract the habit of cigarette smoking. Extreme difficulty was experienced in getting a small part of the sum allocated to discovering what the effects of the advertising campaigns were.

Porter: In the Overseas Development Ministry the amount of money spent on evaluating what we have done has not been large. It is always difficult to persuade people to spend money on this; there is also the fact that we support projects in other people's countries and we have to get their agreement to the evaluation or persuade them to do it, and there may be sensitivities. However, we have now started, and the World Bank has also begun systematically building evaluation systems into on-going projects. We have now an interesting research project, evaluating the effects of a road programme which the ODM is financing in Nepal. The evaluation is designed to look at the effects of the roads on income distribution and changes in industrial and agricultural patterns. We have also financed a consultancy to look at the effects of building a new capital city in Belize. I hope that more of this evaluation will be built into future development projects from the start.

Jones: I am grateful for the reference to my efforts to raise money to evaluate effects of the anti-smoking campaign! It was indeed a desperate effort, and the outcome of the evaluation was rather inconclusive. I am worried about evaluation; it's a nice round term, and all quasi-real scientists would like to know what they have achieved. But behaviour change is very difficult to assess. In absolute terms, to use the example of cigarette smoking, it is relatively easy to measure the total amount of tobacco smoked per head per year. What comes before a behaviour change is an alteration in attitude to tobacco smoking, just as a change in public attitude towards the placing of a particular industry laid out in a particular way is a measure of a general change of attitude. Whether the money required to measure these changes (which could be transient, and subject to fashion) is worth spending until we have a clear picture of the indices we are going to use in the evaluation, I don't know. I am doubtful about the validity of measurements of attitude change and behaviour change.

Murray: Dr Gilson made a good point about quantifying the effects of industrialization. The only place where there has been a positive effort to measure this is in Yugoslavia where Olga Maček, a physician, looked at an area that was about to industrialize. She made studies before industrializing, and is continuing the study during the industrializing operation[1].

The other point is the difficulty of evaluation. I have looked at Teesside over the last 13 years and what is difficult to measure is the 'feel' that Mr Challis mentioned: the fact that there is a greater sense of identity about this area now than 13 years ago. This may be partly because Teesside is now officially recognized as an entity and no longer as a series of discontinuous towns, but I am aware of a sense of civic pride which extends right into the factory. Industrial relations, for example, in the factory, are very much better than 10–15 years ago.

Illich: We have come together here to evaluate the impact of industrial environments on health and to try to discover what the health profession can do about it. The modern medical environment is certainly *part* of the industrial environment. Hospitals, for instance, must be considered as part of the industrial environment for health care, and the hazards of hospitalization, the hazards of increasingly more institutionalized and more technical health care, the hazards of the technification of intervention—of engineering intervention into people's lives for the sake of supposedly increased health, and in people's environments for this purpose—constitute another area of industrial hazard. Is this a legitimate part of our study of industrial health?

As a layman, what I find in terms of medical studies on this point is quite surprising. The Under-Secretary of State for Health of the US claims that 7% of all people discharged from US hospitals in 1971 had legitimate and well-documented grounds for seeking restitution for torts which happened as a consequence of accidents and of involuntary malpractice, and that the accumulated value of these claims was the equivalent of about five times the money spent on the cure of these people. Thus half the hospital budget of the US would have to go for undoing torts, in the narrow legal sense, resulting from industrial environments supposedly intended for health care.

Dickinson: I have been trying to integrate some of the points made here in my own mind. I find that, first of all, we are all in favour of industrialization to some degree; we believe there are lessons to be learnt from the industrialization process we have gone through in western societies, and that in western societies the purely economic good must be replaced by a more human view of the design and purpose of industry. We are trying to suggest to developing countries that they set up industries suited to their own social and productive needs. Such industries would not necessarily be copies of ours. They should be encouraged to look to our industries for lessons on social benefit rather than as sources of hardware that may be copied uncritically. We are also suggesting that they have great advantages to gain by dealing with local raw materials and resources rather than copying the resource use patterns of different societies in other parts of the world. We believe that their industrial medicine should be preventive rather than curative, and that they have much to learn from the social and economic disadvantages, of our approach to both industry and medicine.

We have also looked critically at our predictive capacities and have recognized the important lessons of the building of the Volta Dam at Akosombo. This is an instance where we have a chance of learning a lot about prediction and about ourselves and we shouldn't ignore it. As Lord Ashby has suggested, we should try to see whether we would still make the same mistakes even if we were able to predict events more accurately.

We have now moved to the idea of evaluation, which rapidly becomes 'how do we evaluate evaluation?' This seems to be the key point, and more important than the question of what kind of evaluation we use. Even if we set up fairly arbitrary criteria of evaluation between two different sets of objectives, or between two approaches to the same set of objectives, it doesn't mean that anyone else can understand our evaluation unless we share a considerable background of common experience with them. We are beginning to approach an overall concept of industrialization through the common factors of energy use and resource availability rather than accepting a narrowly economic overview. We might then postulate a unit of energy for such comparisons, but this does not provide us with any common evaluation features in human terms.

White: I like Professor Papanek's idea that we should throw knowledge open to everyone and that his schemes should be made freely available. One of the main reasons why there is concentration of wealth in the world and, therefore, so little development in the poor countries, is because information at many levels is monopolized. Even in medicine this happens, where doctors want to be the only people who can provide medicine. In education too, people institutionalize the giving out of education through certificates of completed education and so on—a point that Ivan Illich has taken much further.

I see this same trend to a monopoly of information in the pleas for evaluation being made here. We have been talking about *us*, as experts, trying to find out what people at ground level think about things, what their attitudes are and then asking, as experts, whether it was worthwhile doing something because people wanted it or whether we should have spent the money on something else. Instead, we should be asking Mr Challis to say how much it cost, per worker, to provide the chemical plant with grass and flower beds, so that everyone could compare this sum with the extra wages that the workers could have been paid. And even more important, the community as a whole might be more interested in whether that money could have been better spent on something elsewhere completely different. For instance, what if you had spent the money used to improve the chemical plant on the health of people in the Sahel? Perhaps we, as a world community, if that information was made available, would decide that it was more valuable to save the lives of say 10 000 people in Africa than to give a little more happiness, which is unmeasurable, to some workers on Teesside. That is a deliberately strong way of putting it, because one is accustomed to think in terms of national boundaries, but I think that the Industrial Revolution and the growth of capitalism in Europe have caused the poverty of the Third World and that we *must* think of it in world terms, and not erect national boundaries so that we can feel that we have an egalitarian society because workers on Teesside feel that. We don't have an equal society in the world.

As a separate general point, economists have long assumed that the problem in underdeveloped countries is one of capital accumulation—if you could get more capital accumulated you would get faster development. It is a false problem, because capital is merely embodied labour—the result of work that has been done in the past—and there are ways other than by building up more money in which you can develop. One such way has been discussed here. It is to design new ways of making things, or new things, which can fulfil the functions being fulfilled at present, or fulfil the needs that people can be seen to have, or that they see themselves as having, in new and simpler ways. This is what intermediate technology does. This is relatively acceptable to the politicians who represent élites in various countries because it doesn't harm their interests too much. It may harm a few commercial interests: if you make a battery-case out of bamboo, a commercial interest that has been making them in tin may oppose you. You may even lose a battle or two but you can do something.

The other way of creating capital without forcing savings out of people (which is thought to be involved by classical economists, and by economists of the Soviet Union, who also think that to accumulate capital one must wrest it out of current production), is to organize people so that they use more of the time or effort that they don't now put into work, to create capital by their own activities without being paid for it. The only way to do that is for people to be organized so that they want to work today for something they will reap in the future. That can be done on a large or small scale, but it has to be a form of socialism, namely an organization of people who will not ask for wages today for what they do, but will be prepared to build a dam because in five years they will have higher productivity from their land. It has been suggested that we propose more radical solutions here, and this political question of the need for collective organization is just one way.

Bridger: The problem of communication affects us all. At the present time we have a tower of Babel of specialisms and of different fields of work. The confusion that arises relates not only to differences in language or values between West and East or between one country and another but between the 'cultures' of our professions and disciplines. It is not sufficient just to understand English even when that language is in general use. It has been said that it is seldom the words or the language that are the root of difficulties in communication. It is not infrequently the ideas being transmitted or the 'music' behind the words. We all have experienced this dilemma. For example, the most bitter arguments can arise between those interested in physical psychiatry and those concerned with the psychotherapeutic aspects.

The same applies here. When the subject of evaluation and the question of assessment came up, I was aware that, as a past mathematician, I understood what was wanted and demanded. At the same time, in my present field, I am concerned more with the *process* of evaluation. If we are to avoid building Babel we must learn to evaluate and test with each other—but without the penalty of humiliation, loss of status or career setback. Thirty years ago it was possible to have opportunities in research, in large-scale activities concerned with *war*, that we cannot have now. I have often had the foolish thought that if only we could have a war now without a war! Because in activities where you have an external enemy, it is so much easier to realize that you have to do something about the situation and be prepared to learn from what you are doing. You cannot convince people of this in peace-time, so-called. The Machiavelli principle all too readily comes into play. On the other hand, where the strength of commitment and sense of purpose can be effectively mobilized—at least to make a start—a 'war' effort is achieved. It was Norway which reviewed its national policy in concert between government, employers, trade unions and others in such a way that people have been applying discoveries made in Britain and elsewhere. This particularly related to the years of research done by the Tavistock Institute on understanding the interrelationship and characteristics of social and technical systems; the characteristics of group working under different conditions and with differing objectives and so on. Although originally derived from studies in mining and textiles, the principles have since ranged over all kinds of study in community life—and at all levels in organizational life. Derivatives of this work have led to job design principles, experiments in work structuring and autonomous work groups. A recent survey of the 'state of the art' was conducted by Lisl Klein of the Tavistock Institute for the German Government[2].

At the same time, much progress has been made in understanding the group and work processes operating in task-oriented groups under conditions of uncertainty, complexity and turbulence, externally and internally. This work on groups operating as 'open systems' and needing self-review as part of their effectiveness was first reported in this Foundation's symposium on *Teamwork for World Health*, held at Istanbul in 1971[3].

References

1. See KEARNS, J. L. (1973) *Stress in Industry*, Priory Press, London
2. KLEIN, LISL (1974) New Forms of Work Organisation. Report to the Kommission für Wirtschaftlichen und Sozialen Wandel (The Tavistock Institute of Human Relations, SFP 2949)
3. *Teamwork for World Health (A Ciba Foundation Symposium)* (1971), pp. 186-190, Churchill, London [now Edinburgh]

Influencing individual and public responses

W. T. JONES

The title of this paper may appear to have chilling illiberal overtones, implying the manipulation of the behaviour of individuals and groups of people for nefarious purposes. It is perhaps because this type of manipulation has happened frequently in recent political history that there has been so little exploration of the constructive methods and uses of engaging public interest and participation in matters affecting health.

Traditionally, doctors, scientists and others have first proposed and gone on to dispose of such matters and the majority of the recipients of these—usually beneficial—efforts have been required to passively follow. One of the bases of this paper is that public attitudes and behaviour are changing and at an increasing pace. No longer are the better educated, the more articulate, the politically active willing to accept unquestioningly the lofty prescriptions of yesterday without accompanying information, explanation, discussion, representation and monitoring. Indeed the full panoply of democratic participation must increasingly be involved when decisions are made about health. In Britain two recent examples of the recognition of these altered circumstances can be seen.

The first is the establishment as a statutory part of the reformed National Health Service of Community Health Councils[1] representing many formal bodies nominated by the Minister from representatives of local opinion, local government, voluntary associations and professional health workers. They are charged to ensure that the administering Health Teams for their local districts are made aware of, and recognize, the health needs of the communities they serve, at least as expressed through the Community Health Councils. Whether in fact representatives of bodies, which are themselves an atypical selection of the population, do accurately reflect the local community's actual needs is hard to say. It is an assumption in our democracy that the chairmen of the local

203

parish council, the local trades council and so on can do this and, once they have such a representative role, it is also presumed that they can go on to identify, interpret and transmit to authority the health needs of the local population. A basic tenet of our democracy in the UK is that one elects a local councillor or Member of Parliament and he then represents our overall interest in all issues; but we know that M.P.'s in particular are determined to follow their own path once they are elected, especially in matters of conscience, so their ultimate effectiveness in voicing the true needs of the community remains to be observed. Public attitudes are changing so rapidly in favour of participation in decision-making that the Community Health Councils had to be introduced into the very core of decision-making in the National Health Service.

As a second example, the new Health and Safety at Work Act 1974[2] fundamentally depends, within the workplace, upon the informed and active participation of representatives of the employees in the day-to-day implementation of its provisions. These employee representatives have statutory authority and responsibilities and seem to represent the beginnings of participation by employees in one section of the general functions of the management of their places of work. How effective these ventures will be in practice again remains to be seen. Perhaps in the small community of a factory, where informal communication at all levels of the hierarchy is better than in the more diffuse world of the domestic community, the representatives, who will probably be the shop stewards, may be truly representative. The British institution of shop stewards is often maligned by those who don't know what a shop steward does, and some more objective observers think that only saints—or power maniacs— become shop stewards, because it is such a demanding job. The shop steward is nobody's friend and everybody's butt; he is ground between the many sectional vested interests of his constituents, and yet has to represent a consensus. For the most part, shop stewards are truly representative of the people they represent (if they are not, they can be got rid of in the next shift). So the new form of participation under the new Act may represent more effectively the views and needs of the factory community.

Both of these new institutions were called into existence by political action and are the result of an underlying demand by the public to be closely involved when decisions are made affecting health. Indeed, there already had been ominous signs that the pre-existing non-participatory institutions were becoming not only ineffective but counter-productive.

The second base of this paper is the obverse of this coin. Participation, to be effective, must be founded upon knowledgeable and motivated participants. There are difficulties here in the health field, part historical and part inherent to the matter itself. For the ordering of the daily affairs of life most societies have evolved, particularly at community levels, systems of representation which take decisions on behalf of the body corporate that are by and large acceptable to it and are implemented for it. Part of the present demand to participate in health matters comes from this root. Another root is the realization, perhaps through the wider and longer education of recent generations, that the mysteries of medicine and science can be adequately penetrated by lay people to allow sufficient understanding upon which intelligent participation can be based. Added to these is the realization, of late, that life and health are no longer chance advantages acquired by a fortunate few but can largely be predetermined by personal choice and communal behaviour allied to knowledge.

A newer root can be detected in some wealthier societies. In places it is being recognized—and Illich[3] has already mentioned this—that a fruitful half century or so of medical and scientific discovery may be closing. Some more recent applications of new knowledge have been less than successful because of unforeseen complications involving ecological balance, the drain on natural resources and the unanticipated contrariness of human behaviour. Scepticism about these events has led to proposals being made for a return to a greater degree of personal responsibility for the everyday details of health and life based upon an acceptance of some of its inevitabilities, such as discomfort, grief, death, about which medicine can do little and the individual can do more. Perhaps individuals are coming to see that they can often do as well, or better, when left to their own means and devices. But inevitably the realization carries with it an increasing demand to participate in decisions that relate to health.

Nevertheless, the dominant historical factor in all of this is the almost universal absence at all levels of any prior experience of lay people in participation in the regulation of fundamental health affairs. The health professions still retain the exclusiveness of the medieval guilds and lay people have been discouraged from prying. Increasingly, fewer people are willing to passively accept the proposals and prescriptions of the professionals without demur; but often their knowledge is scanty and their motivation becomes distorted by malcommunications, and so mutual suspicions follow. Beginnings must be made to correct these deficiencies with due speed or avoidable, unnecessary and unproductive confrontations will increase. As a start the professions must become less exclusive about information to which individuals require access as of right, as well as expediency.

The way to reduce this exclusiveness of the medical professionals would seem, at first glance, in these days of the mass communications, to be straightforward. The television screen, the transistor radio, increasing literacy, the ready availability of the printed word and the development of propaganda techniques would seem to make it relatively easy to impart information, to increase the motivation of people wishing to participate, and to further people's competence to do so. We know from bitter experience that this is not so, or the rate of consumption of tobacco in the UK would be falling rapidly, and there would be an overwhelmingly successful programme of family planning in India. Mass communications are in fact a very limited tool. The advertisers are gratified by a 10% public response to their efforts at specific changes in human behaviour on single concrete issues at a single point in time—such as the sale of a new soap powder. Of course, they hope that this behaviour change will go on to produce a second type of response, namely a continuing, sustained change in behaviour, leading people to continue to buy the product. This should be the aim in our approach, as doctors, to lay people. Whether it is to encourage participation or to influence health behaviour, we cannot be satisfied with the once-for-all response to the type of educational campaign that has been mounted up to now, such as the campaigns encouraging immunization and mass radiography. These are examples of the once-only type of individual-response campaign, and they are largely archaic in conception. The problems are now of altering, in a sustained way, behaviour affecting diet, cigarette smoking, alcohol consumption, drug abuse. When daily life becomes oppressive, people must be prepared not to reach for a cigarette as a prop or to forget the pill, and must be prepared by us to sustain their behaviour change. Unfortunately, we don't know how to do this.

The health professions must not put their trust in the mass media alone; they are an imperfect tool, just as a stethoscope alone is inadequate for diagnosing a heart condition. That television or the mass media generally will achieve sustained behaviour changes is a facile notion.

The public desire to participate in health matters must be matched by increasing knowledge and motivation and the process must begin with the health professionals, who possess the information.

It is in the context of the subject of this symposium—health and industrial growth—that the public demand to be involved has had some of its most dramatic expressions. For example, a cursory glance at the annual reports of many manufacturing corporations will reveal the strength of this feeling and the impact that it has had upon the dealings of men who frequently can remain aloof from such strictly non-business affairs.

Experiences with the Volta Dam Project in Ghana have demonstrated how often health issues are interwined with matters of ecology and environment. Other areas of public concern have centred retrospectively on public disasters, like that of Minamata Bay in Japan or the recent (1974) explosion in Great Britain at the caprolactam plant at Flixborough. An official Inquiry is being held into this latter disaster, and this represents a form of public participation. Britain has other, fairly limited forms of participation: Lord Ashby's Royal Commission on the Environment was a form of public participation. But an inquiry such as that into the disaster at Flixborough is an *ad hoc* procedure, and there has been some controversy over the idea that parts of such inquiries should be held in private because of the secret and confidential nature of the technology of the industrial processes. Secrecy about a business that has already led to 29 deaths and to massive destruction around the plant is unacceptable to some who believe that the company has forfeited any right to continuing confidentiality; more importantly, it is felt that any secrecy in the Inquiry may invalidate its findings and discredit it. A recent letter to *The Times* (13th September 1974) expressed this point of view.

In Britain the Royal Commission on Environmental Pollution offers permanent machinery for a continuing, two-way public response but, outside this, only overtly political machinery and methods are available. Perhaps increasing public knowledge and involvement will mean that existing institutions will adapt to meet these newer needs, but the increasing number of sectional pressure groups concerned with narrow specific issues, often of transitory, local importance, suggests that the adaptation of existing bodies may be too slow. There would seem to be a real danger that poor understanding by the public of the health implications of industrial growth, particularly over specific local issues, such as the effect of a large airport on local inhabitants, may paralyse necessary expansion. Not all industrial growth is harmful, as it is often at present presumed *prima faciae* to be. Indeed the greater good to a larger population, even across international boundaries, can often become obscured by local and narrower interests.

The provision of adequate information to encourage more knowledgeable public responses is often profoundly difficult. Often the long-term biological effects of the new products, the processes involved, and the effluents they produce are not known and are literally unpredictable. Full disclosure of medical and scientific ignorance can feed the alarm of the public, who feel exposed to these hazards, and their alarm is often reinforced by a combination of past failures, bad communications and low levels of basic education. The dilemma here is acute and to some extent is sharpened by the contrast between the immediate benefits that science can bring and the later uncertainties about effects on health. Frequently this is all compounded by a failure, at least in the public eyes, of the professionals to disclose frankly their doubts and anxieties about the future. How much of the current public suspicion of the 'experts' is due to these failings is impossible to estimate. The future should see an increasing willingness by them to enlist public understanding by providing better and freer information. This will in time reduce the level of scepticism but the dilemma of what to say, at what time and in what way, so that all-round integrity remains, and is seen to remain, intact is still unresolved. At least an earlier and closer involvement of public representatives in matters raising general concern over health should give them, and perhaps their constituents, an insight into, and a responsibility for, decision-making.

Ironically, it appears that the larger environmental-cum-community threats of industrial growth have set the pace for a late upsurge of interest by organized labour in work-related threats to health. Interest by employees in the cruder matters of physical safety and health at work has for two decades tended to be lower than comparable interest in, say, road safety or the safety of consumer goods. At a more sophisticated level only rarely, until of late, have the longer range hazards from, say, dusts and noxious fumes been of wide interest[2]. Although concern about occupational health and safety is rising rapidly over the more traditional risks, it is rising faster where long-term carcinogenic effects and pulmonary fibrogenesis are involved. Often the degree of alarm about newer hazards is statistically disproportionate when compared to older, better-documented risks. Such is our ignorance about the influencing of human behaviour that the priorities of medical care can become badly distorted as a consequence of such gusts of interest. Whatever the origins of this recent and welcome phenomenon, the effects on public responses have been similar to those in the community at large. Increasingly, employees are requiring to be informed about the effects on health of the introduction of new processes and of alterations in existing procedures. Acceptance of the risks of familiar work is being less readily given and increasingly questioned.

It is not unknown for industrial physicians to be presented with demands from their employees for the closure, suspension or modification of a process that people have 'known' about for many years and about which they have now become 'aware', often through a misunderstanding of the limited information available to them. The biggest single common factor in these sorts of exaggerated requests is lack of information. It is very rare for people who are provided with all the information that is available, and with a comprehensible interpretation of it, to make a misjudgement. We, as professionals, have been condescending in our attitudes to what people can understand about complex issues. Are we frightened to give all the information in case it is misinterpreted and we shall have to disentangle some malresponse? In my experience, the reverse happens: the more information is given, provided that it is presented in an understandable form, including frankness about uncertainties and lack of knowledge, the more lay people respond in a rational way. Often earlier misunderstandings, which have aroused emotions by overdramatic presentation of limited information, have to be undone, but if the information is presented properly, a rational response is the more usual outcome. It is easier to formalize channels of communication in industry than in society as a whole, because of the hierarchical structure. Channels of communication must of necessity already exist in an industrial concern—the channels by which orders are given and responses received—and these channels can be used for the communication of information, and for participation as well.

Time-honoured agreements about working practices are now being questioned, and management are under increasing pressure to become accountable for them to a broader public. Of late, in Britain and elsewhere, statutory provision has been made to establish methods which will allow employees to participate actively in decision-making. How effective these provisions will be seems to depend upon the level of knowledge of the employees, as well as the managerial participants, and upon how motivated both parties are for making an unfamiliar system effective. There is little scientific understanding of how human behaviour can be influenced in such situations. There are many successful experiments and many unsuccessful ones. Trial and error may need to be the basis in the initial stages. Modern management methods can help with the procedures, and the education and training of the participants is equally important, but guaranteed and repeatable effective and positive responses will be unlikely for some years.

Sir Thomas Legge, who was Dr Murray's predecessor as Medical Adviser to the TUC and Chief Inspector of Factories, about fifty years ago, noticed the fact that human beings are often irrational, unpredictable, contrary, and frequently a bit of a nuisance, particularly to administrators. He was so sceptical about influencing human behaviour that he developed an approach to employee safety which virtually said that only as a last resort would he allow any person to have any control over the protection of his own health at work. Every bit of machinery had to be enclosed, guarded, cut off from the employee as a means to protect him because, Legge implied, he was unpredictable. Therefore, only in the last resort would he provide the worker with a safety helmet or a pair of safety shoes or a mask to wear on his own volition. Times have changed. I am not sufficiently optimistic to think that Legge may not still be largely right, but what has happened is that industrial growth has brought the need in many industries for a better-educated employee. If a complicated plant is to work, the employee has to be better educated than was his father and with this comes a demand to be better informed about the nature of the work. This increasing awareness by the employee is at the root, in industry, of the increasing demand to participate. The health professions still hold the key to much of this, but no longer do we hold it alone.

Discussion

Dickinson: I would like to comment on your point that the mass media don't really get through to people. The mass media face the same problems as the promoters of religious conversion: there is a weak-minded section of any community that can be sold anything, but the reason that people in the main appear resistant to the point of bloody-mindedness is that they are bloody-minded only in terms of *your* grouping, *your* factory, *your* bureaucratic society or parliamentary constituency, or *your* religious sect. But real people don't live in these groups. There are subcultural groups within industry and everywhere else where people live and work together and in which they have their own ground rules which are fully understood, within the group. People are rational within the terms of these groups. It is no use complaining that people are difficult; this only means that you have invented a group which doesn't exist, playing a game to your rules, which are unknown to them. Until you can get through to the real subgroups in any society, whether tribal or industrial, you can have no participation; when you do get through to these groups, the speed at which things happen can be amazing.

Bridger: I agree with Mr Dickinson. There are some examples that are illuminating here. During the war a large experiment was done in the US on changing food habits, in which the approaches of advertising were compared with what happened when people were influenced by explanations and discussions in their own institutions, the work place and the ordinary social groupings within their communities[4]. Efforts were made to discover how best to persuade Americans to eat more brown bread and other foods. The evidence was measurable and significant but has hardly been used, in a full sense, since. A similar experiment was also carried out on National Bonds by the same group. Interaction and commitment based on 'own' decisions, when the group grew to 'own' the problem and formulate their own solutions, led to longer retention of changed behaviour than occurred through the use of advertising and other similar exhortative or persuasive techniques. Since that time, group dynamics and socio-technical systems have enlarged our horizons. Recently we had a wonderful opportunity in the UK to apply some of the research developments of the war and the last 30 years in the reorganization of the National Health Service. As a member of an Area Health Authority, I know the heavy price paid by all the professions, administrations and others in having to make a structure work which neglects so much knowledge and experience. Both the structure and the way it was implemented reflects no credit on Elliott Jaques and his team at Brunel University or on McKinsey and the Department of Health. A closed system of pseudo-consultative groupings has only demonstrated again the penalty for seeking intellectual compromise solutions where neither value systems nor power and authority issues could be imported and reflected upon by those concerned. The result is a case study of a travesty of organizational change conducted by three bodies each rooted in concepts, standards, norms and values of their own: Brunel rooted in the Glacier Metal Company project (the relevance to the NHS is difficult to envisage), McKinsey rooted in current business management practice, and the Department rooted in Civil Service and bureaucratic practice. In themselves each has its importance to the 'owning' institution, but the resulting patchwork is being paid for in great personal, professional and administrative stress.

Phoon: I entirely agree with Dr Jones that the medical profession has been too much of a priestly hierarchy in different forms for many hundreds of years, and younger members of many of the professions in my part of the world have been leading a movement to get rid of this image and to get more participation by lay people and by people from the other professions. We have set up the Singapore Professional Centre, in which social scientists, engineers, doctors and economists can come together to discuss problems facing our society. Each particular society surely needs to select its own solutions from a range of options, but these solutions cannot be worked out on a uni-disciplinary basis, but require the collaboration of all disciplines and sectors of the population.

In the medical profession we have tried to do various things. I have spent much time recently writing a book for schools on what we call 'Human and Social Biology'. I feel it is worthwhile to start teaching people how to live at the level of the schools and even the kindergarten. We have also been producing films for the educational television service so that people can see what is happening to their own country: changes in the ecology, health developments and so on.

We are fortunate in many South-East Asian countries, including Singapore, to have community centres or their equivalent. In the villages we try to inculcate knowledge about health matters through the Head Man or *penghulu*. It is often better to speak to him and let him then talk to the people in front of you, rather than speak directly to them; people listen to the *penghulu*, who commands much prestige. In a way he is something like a shop steward! He has to have this measure of popularity to retain his job as a *penghulu*. In Singapore we do not have so many *penghulus* but we have community centres throughout the island and doctors and other health workers go to them to speak on health subjects. Where necessary, we train people to speak the appropriate dialect. We have had some success in getting rid of the mystery surrounding medical matters, among even the less sophisticated people in South-East Asia.

On industrial health, our new measures on health and safety include full participation by employees on safety committees. A few years ago I suggested the idea and was met with a lot of resistance by managers, who said people would use these opportunities to press wage claims, but it has not been so, and now by law factories of a certain size must have safety committees with representation by the workers.

Lawther: I want to come to the defence of my two heroes, Sir Thomas Legge and the British working man, and to question Dr Jones' interpretation of Legge's fifth aphorism. I don't think Sir Thomas Legge was implying any contempt for the working man's intelligence or underlining his bloody-mindedness in emphasizing that the means of protection must be beyond the control of the worker. I think his aphorism contains an implicit rebuke to ourselves. We have all seen men unwisely discard their masks. This could be attributed to them just being silly and not taking advice; but we do not recognize the complexity of the processes of thought that lead us to give this advice. We ought not to interpret the aphorism as saying that such men are so stupid that one can't trust them with anything; rather we may underestimate the complexity of our own education and our failure to explain the underlying processes. Wherever an effect and its cause are grossly separated in time it is difficult to persuade a man to take precautions. The danger about nitrous fumes, so-called, is that they are not very irritating to breathe, and even physicians don't know why 12 hours after inhalation a person may develop pulmonary oedema and drown; so how can we expect somebody without knowledge of chemistry or physiology to report to the ambulance room or put a mask on when he smells such fumes? We have to remind ourselves that we can never be laymen again, and that we have acquired knowledge the complexity of which we take for granted; maybe we should do a bit more humble education at the work place.

Murray: The axiom was concerned with responsibility: that the primary responsibility is with the employer, and only when he has fulfilled his responsibility can you expect the worker to undertake his. I have been impressed with this in engineering works where there is a problem of serious noise which it is at present impossible to eliminate. The men have accepted the need to wear hearing protection, because there is no alternative, in order to continue with their jobs. I agree with much of what Dr Jones said, particularly the increasing sophistication of workers. I had an example of this in a dispute at the lead-smelting refinery in Avonmouth. This arose primarily because the doctor refused to tell the men their blood lead levels. I spoke to the doctor, who said that you don't tell a patient what his blood pressure is, or it might alarm him. I said that these men drive motor cars: they may not understand the chemistry of the breathalyser test but they know that if it shows more than

80 milligrams alcohol per 100 millilitres of blood they are drunk, however they feel. Equally they can understand that if they have more than 80 micrograms of lead per 100 millilitres of blood, there is a problem. The worker today is sophisticated and one has to take account of this. Nonetheless, we have to interpret for the worker the significance of our figures. It is not always easy; I talk about the calculated risk, and there is a difference between the epidemiological attitude to the frequency of disease in the population and the individual attitude about the disease of a certain person. When I talk about the calculated risks, they say 'That's all right for you, doc; you make the calculations; we take the risks!'

Challis: What is needed in dealing with people is human understanding, and while it is right to set up systems and have safety organizations and safety committees, and it is right for there to be an exchange of views on health and so on, the thing which frees the human blockage is whether the people listening trust you or not, and this is a hard test. It is something which is not easily subjected to analysis and something from which most technical men in industry tend to shrink. I make this point because I have some sympathy with Mr Illich's paper, which made a big impact on me. It is right that we talk about management systems, but we must remember as technical people not to overlay the system so that it becomes a thing in itself. The working man today in the West is very well educated compared to his father and that education means that he can grasp concepts much wider than people think, particularly technical people. You have to use the local language, and to use some sensitivity and ask yourself, if you were on the other side, what you would like to know. And since we are all human, we *can* ask ourselves that, and get a feeling for it. I am talking from my own area of knowledge, which is not medical, but I suspect that it is relevant to the medical profession too.

Ramalingaswami: Dr Jones gave us an important message for medicine; this is *the* area of unfulfilled expectations in medicine[5]. We have hospital medicine; we have environmental activities such as DDT spraying, but done without the participation of people. But there is a third area, a large gap between what medicine can do and what it is doing, between the needs of individuals in the environment of their homes and farms and the capabilities of modern medicine. Its proportions are truly gigantic in the developing world, and *the* challenge for the future.

The modern physician is often in a helpless position when he starts to talk to people about their illnesses; how do you explain influenza to a rural person? But this is done beautifully by the local indigenous physician, because the language, the culture, the mould, are all those that such people are familiar with; they use traditional and familiar terms. This adaptation of medicine and medical terminology to the level of understanding of people is the dimension in medicine which is most neglected. Health education has become hackneyed. Often there is much concern for the medium and less for the message. The casting of the message within the framework of the people you are communicating with is the crucial problem.

Ashby: This relates to the question of the 'exporting' of ideas from the West, which has come up several times already. One of the most suspect exports from the developed countries, particularly the UK, has been higher education. In the 1850's we exported higher education to India and started three universities. Nothing was done to safeguard what are called 'standards'. The remoteness from London University (which was the model), and the fact that the new universities were composed by the federation of large numbers of colleges already there, prevented this. One remembers the terrifying statement of Macaulay that he wanted to create in India a class of persons Indian in blood and colour, but English in tastes, in opinions, in morals and in intellect. This was the basis of the British policy. But attempts to bring early graduates up to the standard of graduates from British universities were disappointing. In 1900 the failure rate reached 75%. Thereafter standards were settled locally and they fell, so much that when Queen Victoria died a leader in the *Calcutta Times* suggested that, in deference to the Queen Empress, the university should lower the pass rate by 25% that year! This failure to attach its degrees to an international standard has been one of the great embarrassments in Indian higher education; it is being overcome slowly but with difficulty now.

In the 1950's, a hundred years later, the British started exporting universities to Africa, and one of the decisions was not to repeat that mistake; instead of which they made another mistake that was just as bad. It was decided to give a degree to the new African universities which would be a facsimile of a London University degree.

We are concerned here with the effects of this on medicine. I was involved in the beginnings of some of these African universities and, having seen at first hand the Soviet system of medical service, I pleaded for something comparable to the *feldsher* system in the USSR. There, besides doctors trained to as high a standard as anywhere in Europe, able to do specialist work and provide hospital services, there are also large numbers of medical assistants. Some enlightened British medical professors were in favour of a similar system in tropical African countries, but this was contemptuously dismissed by the more pedantic of my colleagues as a 'lowering of standards'. It would not have been a lowering of standards; it would have been the introduction of a new coin in the medical currency, which is quite a different matter. However, my impression now of some African countries, although they are recovering from the mistakes in our 'export policy', is that they still favour the production of highly sophisticated doctors in sophisticated medical schools, whose main object is to stay in the cities and to look after the hernias of cabinet ministers rather than to disseminate public health measures such as the designing of earth closets in villages. I cannot urge too strongly that countries developing health services and still with room for manoeuvre will take their courage in their hands and start, side-by-side with Western medical education, a training for a subprofessional medical service to serve in rural areas.

The situation was even worse in veterinary sciences. When I was familiar with these matters (it may be different now) it was impossible to practice in Nigeria unless you had qualifications enabling you to look after cats and dogs in London. This was nonsense in a country where veterinary science was desperately needed in order to improve human nutrition. I feel that we have been in a dilemma. We have done good things to Africa, in exporting a high standard of learning as we know it in our universities. But at the same time, in certain professions, particularly medicine, we have made serious mistakes.

Ramalingaswami: This precisely is the evil of medical education now in India, which is equally a reflection of certain developments in the past. What is interesting, in addition to what you have said, is that there did exist in India a licentiate system during the British period. The candidates were recruited after 10 years of school on the specific understanding that they would spend three years in medical school and then work in a rural setting. They went to the rural areas and many of them did well there. When we became independent, the idea grew that you cannot have a 'second rate' doctor caring for the rural areas; you can't have castes among doctors. So we abolished systematically the schools that had been training licentiates; in addition, those holding the diplomas were enabled to come back to the university for further study for two or three years in the classical hospital setting in order to qualify for a university degree. We are now wondering whether to reintroduce this category again, or something else functionally of a similar type in its place. Such thinking is going on in many parts of the world now. The step we have already taken is to slow down or stop setting up new medical colleges of the type we already have, during the next five years.

The question of international standards in medical education is relevant to our discussion. One often hears the statement made about a new medical school in a developing country, that it will have the standards of Harvard or Johns Hopkins. The highest standards are those most relevant to the particular country or region in terms of the service they can provide. There could be a core curriculum, the grammar of medicine, that could be common across countries.

Dickinson: I take it that the corollary to the loss of the licentiate was the loss of medical services to villages? The qualified doctors don't go to the villages any more?

Ramalingaswami: They do, but not to the extent they are needed.

Holland: I entirely agree with Mr Dickinson. The problem surely is how to persuade graduates who have spent their student years in universities with excellent living accommodation to return to work in their home areas where they will certainly be without running water, electricity and other facilities. I believe the same point was made in Tanzania, the only country which began a new medical school on the basis of recommendations by Titmuss, Abel-Smith, Macdonald and Wood. Unfortunately, the local people, particularly the graduates, refused to accept that their qualifications were different and unacceptable according to the criteria of the USA or the UK.

Derban: Ghana is thinking about the possibility of a second medical school. In the present medical school, as in most medical schools in developed countries, the philosophies of medical care and the education of health personnel focus on high-quality care of individual patients. The educational system based on these philosophies does not therefore fit the needs of the developing world, as has already been pointed out.

The challenge for medical education in Ghana is not to maintain international standards in medical education but to develop and operate a system of health that can bring better care to large numbers of people on limited resources.

El Batawi: It is the policy of WHO to adapt medical and public health education to the local needs of regions and countries. But this should not compromise the level of knowledge the physician should have. It is possible that we can build up programmes of education for health assistants, but once we talk about doctors, it is important not to lower the level of knowledge the physician should have, so he may be able to diagnose, treat and prevent human disease. We may, for example, emphasize tropical medicine in the tropics and emphasize certain aspects in medical sciences, depending on the geographical pathology.

Illich: Dr El Batawi wants doctors who can cope with sickness, but I thought that coping was the basic sign of *health* of individuals. This is also an export—when we export schools we export not only an explicit programme but also a hidden curriculum, namely that schooling from now on is a requirement and a necessity, and therefore learning outside school becomes ugly, autodidactic incompetence; that learning is measurable and one can grade people according to the learning they have acquired on the pyramid of drop-outs which I described earlier; and that certification is an activity of the central government, connected with consumption from the knowledge stock, through people who are holders of knowledge stock certificates.

Norway was mentioned. Niels Christie there leads the battle which aims to make certification by educational institutions illegal. This is not a minority proposal; it is not unlikely that it will pass through parliament in a couple of years. It would limit certification to a very few competences which a special government agency will administer, always on a temporary basis. Milton Friedman, who politically takes a very different position from Christie, suggests that, at least in the US, doctors have acquired so many claims to competence that licensure becomes meaningless, and therefore it should be discontinued and people should be allowed to shop around for their doctors, and then probably most of the disadvantages which are a consequence of licensure could be done away with. Is it not possible to export, at least for discussion purposes, to very poor countries the highest level disappointments and countermeasures proposed in the rich countries at this moment?

Porter: We have covered a very wide area in this question of health problems associated with development, and we should not forget that there are specific hazards associated with particular industrial processes, and similarly in agriculture, with the health hazards now emerging there as a result of the use of pesticides. That is one group of problems which has implications for the training given to medical personnel. There is another order of medical problems arising from urbanization itself, which is *associated* with industrialization, but goes on autonomously: if people just go into cities (and industry is a relatively small proportion of the activity of cities) there is a new range of health problems associated with urbanization. This is another area requiring special techniques and ways of looking at problems, and a special kind of training.

There doesn't seem much point in philosophizing about what *ought* to be: Mr White said we should have socialism throughout the world, but it is surely presumptuous to prescribe to people the social organizations they ought to have. People have to evolve them for themselves. If one is reflecting on this problem and trying to help the process on—say, trying to design systems of training health workers—one needs a vision of where we are now and the likely pattern of development over the next 10–20 years. One can say with some certainty that in many countries a large proportion of the working population is engaged in agriculture at a low level of productivity, they are often widely scattered populations, and there is a major problem of how to deliver health services to them; what measures do you have to take in order to improve the health of that very large population, bearing in mind that improvement in physical standards may be a key to improved productivity, which is an absolute essential? We need to analyse the problem and to identify in each country the endemic diseases which need to be concentrated on.

One can also predict that urbanization will continue and at an increasing rate. There is no apparent force, unless physical violence is used, that will change this momentum, which arises from demographic factors; the people have already been born who are going to live in these cities. There is, therefore, another enormous area of public health problems in urbanization; how does one get to grips with this sort of problem? Is it simply a question of more resources or is it a question of barefoot doctors? If one looks at the problems in this way it might be possible to identify what needs to be done in particular areas to help desperately poor countries, with very limited resources, to cope with these intractable problems, without saying that they ought to have this or that sort of social organization, which is a question for *them*. One has to offer help in this spirit in the context of their own social and economic environment and consistently with their own aspirations and perceptions.

References

1. DEPARTMENT OF HEALTH AND SOCIAL SECURITY (1974) *Democracy in the National Health Service*, DHSS, London
2. *Health and Safety at Work etc. Act* (1974) Chapter 37, HMSO, London
3. ILLICH, I. (1974) *Medical Nemesis: The Expropriation of Health*, Calder & Boyars, London
4. LEWIN, K. (1947) Group decision and social change. In *Readings in Social Psychology* (Newcomb, T. M. & Hartly, E. L., eds.), Holt, Rinehart & Winston, New York
5. RAMALINGASWAMI, V. (1968) Unfulfilled expectations and the Third Approach. *British Journal of Medical Education 2*, 246-248

A social anthropological approach
to health problems in developing countries

GERALD MARS

This paper may not give answers to the problems we have been discussing, but will perhaps suggest some of the right questions. I shall begin by briefly outlining some distinctive features of anthropology; I shall then discuss some of the problems found within innovative organizations, and conclude by suggesting a strategy that might aid innovation.

Anthropology has three features that could be useful in the context of health care in developing countries. Firstly, as a special kind of sociology, distinguished by its area and method of study, its method deserves special attention. Anthropological fieldwork depends predominantly upon a method called 'participant observation': this means that the anthropologist goes into a particular community, lives among its people and submerges himself in their society. And though its area of study has traditionally been concerned with small-scale, 'underdeveloped', non-literate societies, this is a tradition which is now changing. Yet it is because these types of societies have not usually had records available that development of the subject has depended, and still depends, on its getting material directly from the people concerned. It is the degree of this emphasis on participant observation, on direct involvement with the people studied, that distinguishes anthropology from other social sciences.

Such emphasis and indeed dependence on a specific type of research method leads us to consider the second feature of anthropology that concerns us. This is the essentially 'micro' and holistic view of much of its subject matter, anthropologists tending to look for the interconnectedness between different aspects of a small society's workings. They are concerned, for instance, to understand the articulation of family and kinship organization with grass-root political power and authority, the relation of these to religious beliefs and practices, and the place taken in all these affairs by the way goods and services are produced and distributed. One result of this is that anthropologists are geared to making a variety of minutely observed 'micro' studies; another is that the contributions of anthropology in the 'macro' sphere lie in relatively broad generalizations. It has been said that the more 'macro' anthropology gets, the less effective it becomes. But among its very broad generalizations are acknowledgements that the dominant organizing features in many societies are not based on contract, as in our type of industrial culture, but on kinship—that is to say, on birth and marriage and on neighbourhood (that is, on proximity and residence). These are factors on which much of the world's social organization hangs and which innovators concerned with the developing world ignore at their peril. But anthropologists are also interested in such areas as the comparative study of social controls, of the distribution of power and authority and of the linkage of small to larger social units, and these take the subject outside its immediate small-scale area of interest. The articulation of local authority roles to outside power structure, for instance, or to bureaucracies, a matter of obvious interest to innovators in the health field, is increasingly regarded as important by anthropologists.

Anthropology's third distinctive feature is an emphasis on avoiding what is called 'ethnocentricity': the mistake of looking at other people's worlds through the eyes of one's own. Archetypally ethnocentric, for instance, was the famous statement of an Englishman on returning from abroad who, when asked how he had found the natives, replied, 'Customs beastly, manners none!' The anthropologist, in contrast, is trained to continually reexamine assumptions derived from his own culture that he takes with him into the society he is studying. This, I would suggest, is one of the most important contributions that anthropology can bring to dealings with developing countries. Like many observations it states the obvious. But the obvious is often the thing on which to concentrate: if nothing else, it is so often overlooked.

I believe that these three tenets of the anthropologist's approach can aid us in anticipating some of the consequences that may derive from any innovation, including schemes to increase health or to reduce illness. We might not be able to avoid future mistakes, or even with the benefit of hindsight to say with certainty what went wrong with, for instance, the Volta Dam Project, some details of which Dr Derban discussed earlier in this symposium (pp. 49–72). But we might, however, through the application of insights derived from our three tenets, be able perhaps to avoid some of the grosser errors.

Let us first briefly examine some cases of unfortunate innovation in the health field. As one example, Foster[1] (p. 107) quotes an instance from Saudi Arabia where a Moslem worker in a machine shop injured his hand in a lathe and was advised by the American foreman to go to the small company hospital where there was a medical officer. The worker refused, left to visit his kinfolk in the desert and then returned several days later to ask for treatment. But this was by then too late; he already had gangrene. The point to note here is that many decisions we regard as being the sole concern of an individual are, in many cultures, only able to be taken by a wider kin group. There are many other examples. Marriott[2] (p. 243) (also mentioned in Foster,[1] p. 107), reported a case from India of a father and brother asking a medical officer for quinine for their respective daughter and sister, ill with malaria. The quinine was given but three days later had still not been used; the girl's aunt had forbidden it. In this culture decisions on the health affairs of women are made by senior female relatives. These are by no means attitudes that are 'backward', 'primitive' or even limited to rural folk. But the misunderstandings they reveal are typical: ethnocentricity occurs whenever cultures meet and these cultural conflicts can cause misunderstanding even among sophisticated members of professional cultures.

I mentioned earlier in discussion (p. 150) my experiences in Newfoundland which, though part of the North American continent, is, or at least was in the early sixties, an almost archetypal underdeveloped country, with birth rates of over 30 per thousand, a subsistence economy and by far the lowest income per head in Canada. The authorities in the provincial capital tried to introduce the idea of cooperatives to coastal fishermen. But these failed. And when the island confederated with mainland Canada in 1949 the Federal Government tried to bring in road-building systems by focussing money through local village councils. This scheme too failed. There were no such councils or cooperatives in existence and in neither case were they easy to get started. This reflects a common situation in many parts of the world; a refusal of people to adopt leadership roles. It often becomes difficult to focus resources, and to use people to channel changes through, if no one will come forward and one doesn't know who to focus on or channel through. This is a problem found particularly in subsistence economies whose members tend to be geared to the idea that the size of the cake is fixed. If anyone is perceived to get advantage from a development or any other scheme, this advantage, whether it is economic or of pure prestige, is believed to be obtainable only through someone else's loss. The result is that one gets an enforced equality and resistance to the idea of innovation. We need to educate our innovators to appreciate this kind of issue.

But even working through real local leaders is often different from working through leaders who *seem* to be leaders. Again our ethnocentric categories can confuse us. It is, for instance, often ignored that a community might not possess a single political leader. There may, however, be one person who decides, say, when to migrate with cattle, another who sorts out disputes, but perhaps only in an advisory way, and a third who helps to arrange marriages. 'Leadership' of these kinds is often different from the type of executive leadership a would-be innovator tends to think is relevant to his plans for innovation—whether these are concerned with health or other spheres of planned social change and whether they occur in rural or urban situations. In advanced industrial economies too, we find that political innovators who ignore local grass-root feelings and opinions and ignore or more often mistake local grass-root leaders are likely to fail. We in the UK are now realizing, for instance, that if we had retained many of our traditional residential districts and had improved these rather than destroying them and building high-rise flats we would now have more viable neighbourhoods—viable both economically and socially. The answers were there if we had asked the people involved—but no-one did! There is little difference in these respects between such action in developing countries and action in advanced industrial countries; both tend to emanate from bureaucracies and to involve a lack of consultation.

With these examples in mind, let us now consider one successful resettlement scheme, resulting from the building of a dam, and compare some features of its planning with the socially less successful Volta project in Ghana.

Dr Derban and the discussants of his paper (pp. 49–72) have already mentioned some of the problems of subsequent migration from the resettlement area which have overcast the technical feat of the dam's construction. I will therefore not elaborate these details here. But in contrast, some of you will have heard of the Papaloapan Valley Resettlement Project in Mexico, described by Foster[3]. In some respects it can be said to be the basis of much of Mexico's modern economy. It was a massive scheme with resettlement placed under the control of an anthropologist, Alfonso Villa Rojas, and a team of anthropological assistants.

Well before any building began, Rojas and his anthropologists made anthropological studies of the communities to be resettled, and they used the holistic model I have described. In this way they obtained data that enabled forecasts to be made of the impact of change on specific aspects of indigenous life and were therefore in positions to suggest ways of minimizing impacts, where possible by transferring these facets of social organization from the original to the new situation. As one instance, the spatial arrangement of villages was found particularly important in arranging ceremonials, alliances, marriages, and various other cooperative ventures. As a result they were able to incorporate at the planning stage a transfer of the original spatial arrangements to the new villages. And in this new situation they advised that houses be built on the old patterns though they were to be built with newer materials that were more hygienic. When resettlement was complete, provision was made for people to return to visit their old homes until their inundation, which served to ease the shock of their move.

As a result of this approach, when resettlement plans were formulated not only were considerable data available but the real opinion-moulders of each community (as against politically appointed nominal leaders) were able to be identified, approached and used as educational spearheads. They were taken to view prospective sites chosen with knowledge of the communities' social organization in mind and final decisions, though focussed through them, were able to be made with community support after community discussion. One result of this type of participative change was that the normal suspicion between rural peasants and urbanites was minimized. Most of the world's peasants, whether Newfoundland fishermen, Mexican farmers or Ghanaian tribesmen, are (rightly) suspicious of anything emanating from towns; in their experience most such contacts have been harmful. Such rural/urban divisions are, of course, not limited to underdeveloped countries. It is always townsmen who tell rural dwellers what to do and what taxes to pay. It is increasingly townsmen who dominate the country, whether their interests are benign and concerned with health innovation or for any other reason. But because, in this instance, change was able to be focussed through key indigenous leaders it could, in effect and to a degree, be dissociated from the suspicious authority of the town.

It is not, however, the town as such that is a source of suspicion; it is that the authority which dominates people's lives in the increasingly integrated economies of the world is also increasingly external to their control or at least to their perceptions, and we are finding that when this happens, things just do not work—unless and until we are able to by-pass our bureaucracies and bring innovator and 'innovatee' meaningfully together.

If we look at the Volta Resettlement Programme it appears that many planning features found in the Papaloapan Project were absent or at best limited. The most serious defect in planning, apart from the lack of meaningful local involvement, followed from a lack of time, and this was related to a lack of finance for social planning which did not become available until after construction had already begun on the dam in 1961.

As David Butcher, the sociologist called in by the Volta authorities very late in the day, observed, 'If expediency sometimes took precedence over the optimal it was because full plans and working drawings for the dam had been completed and engineering work begun before the creation of the Resettlement Office, let alone the investigation of the full social problem'.[4] (p. 28). Even then the early resources allowed were derisory when the total cost of the dam— £70 million—is considered. Only two officers, an Administrative Officer and an Agricultural Officer, were appointed in 1961 and for many months they lacked real authority or financial resources. As the belatedly appointed Resettlement Officer wrote: 'By May, 1962, when dam construction had been going on for 9 months it became apparent that no progress had been achieved on resettlement and there was no co-ordinated programme' (Kalitsi[5], p. 11). It says much for the staff involved that so much was achieved in so short a time: the efforts expended were heroic and the results, considering the constraints, quite outstanding.

With only two years to go before the water's planned rise, decisions had to be made quickly, and this necessarily limited the possibilities of participation. As a result decisions on types of housing and types of farming had to be pre-empted. 'Once the basic objectives on housing and farming had been agreed (sic) the Resettlement Programme was viewed to be carried out in the following logical phases:

   (i) Surveys and Field Studies.
  (ii) Planning and Programming.
 (iii) Development of Houses and Farming.
  (iv) Evacuation.
   (v) Rehabilitation.'

But, as Kalitsi continues,

'In practice, however, for most of the time surveys, field studies, planning, programming, development of houses and farms were going on at the same time. This was necessitated by the pressure to start building and farming early for the evacuees'. (Kalitsi[5], p. 16).

While decisions in the two areas of housing and farming were already and necessarily pre-empted, the surveys and field studies appeared of necessity to be crash exercises in numerical data collection rather than attempts at obtaining data for the systematic analysis of social structures. But even here, though heroically issued and processed by three-week trained students and social workers, much of this data 'arrived too late to be used for planning. For example, if it were known that the settlers would be accompanied by 2954 cattle, 11 600 chickens and 42 000 sheep and goats some arrangement would have been made to cater for them'. (Kalitsi[5], p. 19).

Three features appear to lie behind the success of the Papaloapan Project and to have been absent from the Volta scheme. Firstly, there was adequate time allowed for pre-planning, which preceded actual dam building, and this permitted modifications to be made to the technical structure while this was still at the planning stage. Second and following from this, the basis of such pre-planning was built upon micro-anthropological studies that were centrally coordinated, monitored over at least a year of fieldwork and, most importantly, had time allowed for their analysis at the end of this period. Questionnaire surveys are never an adequate substitute for this type of work. Thirdly, the resettlement was genuinely *participative*; planning was carried out not only *for* the people involved, but *with them*. In this the selection of key leaders within the communities as educators and as points for focussed change was integral to the whole scheme.

I mentioned, in discussing the success of the Papaloapan Project, the importance of relatively dissociating innovative projects from their origin in the towns. But this concept of *dissociation* need not be confined to relations between rural dwellers and urban innovators: it is as usefully applied to all relationships where a group is affected by change that comes to it from outside or from above. Its successful application, as in Papaloapa, however, depends on *participative involvement*, and this is a cornerstone of much of the work at the Tavistock Institute of Human Relations that deals with planned change both in industrial and in non-industrial settings (see, for instance, Bridger et al.[6]).

This brings us to the functioning of organizations. We have learned that an organization's design can be crucial to the success or failure of its programmes. One can in fact design an organization to do its job in such a way as to guarantee its failure. It is unfortunately true that one cannot design an organization that will guarantee success, but there are approaches that can be suggested and pitfalls that can be avoided. One of our main findings has to do with the adaptability of an organization to the dynamism of its environment. When we are concerned with the alleviation of illness and the extension of health care, we are essentially dealing with an organization that has a very wide interface with its environment and which must, therefore, be extremely sensitive and readily adaptable in its dealings with it if it is to be successful in its tasks.

In such an organization, many of the characteristics traditionally associated with organizational structures no longer apply. In particular, the traditional organization can be conceptualized as a closed system. But an organization closely responsive to its environment must essentially be conceived of as an open system—open, that is, to environmental influences. This openness necessarily influences the interrelationships of colleagues within the organization and their relationships with their hierarchy. Here, the role of leader is more concerned with reconciling the claims of and interacting with different aspects of the environment than in a closed system, where the environment is largely given and where he is much more concerned with the coordination and supervision of the work of subordinates. In an open system, on the other hand, subordinates (who are also working within the environment) need to become interdependent in order to coordinate their own activities[7].

For these reasons it is advisable for innovating organizations to have few levels of authority and to have a broad rather than a narrow pyramidal shape. In this way it is easier to encourage lateral communication, cooperation and team building than if an organization is dominated by a tall pyramidal structure with many levels of authority.

But we are not just talking here of subordinates in the ordinary sense of line managers. The kind of subordinates meant here are those who operate at the actual boundaries of innovative health care organizations and who are highly skilled professionals. As well as finding difficulties in coordinating their roles as members of the same groupings, they also face difficulties that arise from the culture of their professions. Medical doctors, for instance, are trained with the idea that life is sacred and that to calculate the relative cost of treatments and to decide on one rather than another, on perhaps economic rather than on medical grounds, is somehow a negation of this training. And economists have only relatively recently come to see that economic growth and the good life are not necessarily immutably entwined. Many agricultural experts also operate within a conceptual framework derived from economics that in its turn is derived from the industrial West. Their concern is often, it appears, to bring increased yields from a given unit of land with less labour. Our professional orientations in many respects provide a barrier to understanding, not only of the overall needs of people in the situations in which they operate, but also in limiting coordination within effective interdisciplinary teams. It is, however, a problem that can be overcome through training and education.

Lord Ashby in his comments on the transfer of universities from Britain to Africa (p. 214) provided a good example of how an ethnocentric professional culture can clash with the needs of the people it intends to serve, not only because of the innovators' perceptual limitations, but also because of the limitations of its beneficiaries. The professional culture in this case was that of British university builders who were particularly concerned to provide the best of British university experience for Africa, but who failed to take adequate account of how it would transplant to the local situation. This was not entirely through the limitations of the innovators; it was as much due to the reference groups of the consumers who wanted to learn Latin rather than Ibo and who would sooner take a course in Tudor history than in their own history. Most African countries have, in many respects, passed this stage of colonial dependence but the moral to be drawn from this experience still applies. Because the African beneficiaries were élites, they had a reference group not based on their local needs: they referred themselves instead to a wider—a world-wide—élite.

A dramatic example of the practical implications of this kind of reference group, in this case one which was held by administrative and medical professionals in Zambia, is provided in a recent paper by Frankenberg and Leeson[8]. Zambia has spent vast resources on an airport, on parliament buildings and particularly on a teaching hospital. But the reference group of the politicians who furthered the policies that led to these undertakings and the staff who were involved, and the advisers—often from the industrial West—who helped to establish them, was that of a world élite, the 'travelling circus' of experts. They were not looking at base level needs or at available resources in terms of these needs. They were not marrying the two by considering a basic health care unit which could take account of local needs, local values and local social structures. Frankenberg and Leeson point out that as many resources were spent on the establishment of this prestigious and quite excellent teaching hospital as would have provided a 'barefoot' doctor service in the Chinese fashion for every community in Zambia.

Of course, the will to bring about changes of this order in the field of political action depends on much more than a knowledge of local needs. But in the face of short-term innovation of schemes directly liable to affect the welfare of whole communities, it seems evident that an innovator's understanding of local needs as well as of social systems and fears is a vital first step. Participative involvement would appear to be an equally vital second step.

This brings me to the suggestion I briefly referred to earlier (p. 67): that the time has now perhaps come for the use of auxiliaries in innovation. There is no reason why the same pressures on resources and staff which brought into being the barefoot doctor scheme in China should not now be exploited in the anthropological field. I suggest that we should now think of innovating through 'barefoot anthropologists' in an attempt to link social reality to social planning.

One fully trained anthropologist could, with the aid of auxiliaries, monitor up to, say, ten small-scale communities (though the idea could as well apply in towns). The advantages are that monitoring would essentially be two-way and that locally based, locally resident and locally involved people would, initially through the professional, be able to inform and thereby, one hopes, be able to modify and influence the policies of innovators. In this way the auxiliary becomes an extension to and indeed a part of the innovating team, but a part that is rooted in the community.

I hope I have been able to demonstrate how the role of the anthropologist might be of use and how, if multiplied through the employment of auxiliaries, this use may be multiplied. If his skills can be developed not only to cover an understanding of social organization on the ground but also to contribute to the self-conscious awareness of organizational complexities and organizational design among his innovating colleagues, then his role might prove doubly useful.

Discussion

Dickinson: I am encouraged to hear comments from a professional that I, as an amateur, have been struggling towards for some time. I would like to back up Dr Mars by giving four examples of the way in which individuals live in a number of independent subcultures and find little difficulty, except in times of stress, in living according to the differing rules of the separate subgroups.

When I was teaching in Wales, an Iraqi student was taken ill; he became violent and withdrawn and had to have psychiatric treatment. It was discovered that the one assurance he wanted was that though he couldn't take the impending examinations he would be allowed to take the supplementaries at a later date, and the medical authorities had an official come from the university to confirm this. Assurance from such a source wasn't good enough for him and they had to send for me, because he indicated that he would only accept me to speak for the university. It turned out that everybody had ignored him at the university, but I had once given him the dressing down of his life for wasting my time and also his own. On this occasion, I was the one person who could communicate something to him and reassure him.

The second case was in China when a colleague was taken ill in Canton with a heart condition and had to go to hospital. Having got him stabilized, at 2 a.m., they called a meeting which consisted of the doctor in charge, the two nurses in charge, the heart specialist from the People's Liberation Army, the leader of our delegation, a doctor in our party, me as the patient's friend, the two cleaners, the old lady who brewed the tea, and a man who had been on the Long March but whose duties now were to put the flowers around the wards. We all had to have a say on treatment, because treatment depends on the integration of all possible medical and social relationships. The only thing they really worried about was that I should telegraph the patient's employer to ensure that his job was secure! They had a view of the behaviour of a bourgeois employer which required action that only I could take. Otherwise it was a conventional division of labour.

The third point is that in the university department in which I work everyone takes responsibility for some minor administrative matter, without having any official position for it. I look after the safety in the department and recently an attempt was made to persuade me to look after security as well. I pointed out that the two are quite impossible to combine. No-one could accept the argument that these two were not related until the point was made that safety depends on persuasion and security on sanction, the different rules of the sub-culture with regard to persuasion and sanction being immediately recognizable.

The fourth example comes from Ghana. I have made several visits to a number of Ashanti villages. In some villages almost all the men are weavers and get fairly regular earnings, which are relatively low, and in the other villages most men are cocoa farmers who receive larger payments, but once a year. I have been trying to look at the way the people in the two sorts of villages spend their money and the relative benefits of the two modes of re-ceiving income. I suspect that expenditure on education and the saving of working capital is better regulated for the villagers receiving a regular income but a lower total annual payment, than for those getting an annual 'bonanza' who tend to spend it on a good party before they sort out their annual payments. Any attempt to introduce alternative employment in the villages will be greatly influenced by the current practices of earnings distribution.

Illich: I want to give an example of how this works politically, to confirm these ideas. In Chile in the sixties the policy for public health was priority for the better feeding of infants in order to cut down infant mortality. Bottle feeding became 'the thing'. One result of this was that in 1960, 6% of mothers did *not* breast-feed their children at the age of one year. In 1972, only 6% of mothers occasionally fed their babies at one year. There was a total reversal. The additional cow's milk necessary for the unrealized human milk would require about 32 000 additional cows, which Chile's pasture cannot support.

El Batawi: I would like to ask Dr Mars when he was last in a developing country, and for how long, and where? Because my impression from his description of workers and people in developing countries is that it is rather out of date. Both Dr Jones and Dr Murray have indicated that workers are now sophisticated. People working in the Sudan or in Saudi Arabia and in many other countries are often well-educated and progressing rapidly. They participate in decision-making. The so-called underdeveloped countries are developing rapidly, and it is perhaps time for western society to start to learn from these countries.

Mars: I would quite agree that the so-called underdeveloped countries are developing rapidly and in fact I believe it to be well *past* the time for western society to learn from these countries. This indeed was one of the messages I hoped to have put across. Too often experts from industrial society and officials in bureaucracies that are derived from industrial society have not learnt and do not and will not learn from the developing societies in which they operate. I think we agree here?

But though workers may be well educated and highly sophisticated there are still cultural and organizational blocks in any society which always limit the ability of one such group to learn from another. This applies as much to and between top level professionals as it does between illiterate tribesmen.

What I was arguing for, on the basis of work derived from Newfoundland and extending over the past 14 years—and on many counts, from birth rates to deficiency diseases, this was until very recently a classically underdeveloped country—as well as from more limited experience in North Africa, is that it is of much more use when innovating in health care or in anything else if you know how to operate through two cultures. These are the culture of the innovating bureaucracy and the culture of the people you are dealing with. And that certainly means learning from the people on the spot.

White: For some time now in anthropology there has been a tension between trying to understand the needs of tribal people or indigenous people, so as to represent them and to get a better situation for them, on the one hand, and on the other hand helping colonialism (at an earlier period) and (now) modernizers and industrializers to cope with problems that they might meet in their programmes of expansion. Dr Mars' comments remind me of the initial responses of anthropologists when in about 1949–1950 economists entering the field of economic development began to ask anthropologists to solve some of the problems they met. This was the period when development was thought to consist of modernizing on the pattern of western industrialization. This period is now over. We have heard much about participation in this symposium, and the emphasis on participation, self-reliance and micro-development seems to be a relatively better answer than the old modernizing answer. I think it is in fact the only section of a better answer that is likely to get accepted and that the other aspect, of socialist development, is what is really needed. However, you are talking about something which does not go even as far as that.

For example, you mentioned what I would call a low-level equilibrium trap. That is, because in a community everybody is jealous of anyone who gets ahead, nobody is allowed to get ahead, so everybody stays at a low level of living. This was thought in the 1950's to be widespread among peasant societies. It is a phenomenon we all know from school, where every child controls every other child so that he shan't become the teacher's favourite. It is a natural human reaction, but it doesn't correspond to the overwhelming response of people to new opportunities. Even peasants from situations where there is a low-level equilibrium trap, when they go to an outside society where they can earn more, become rich, and may return to their indigenous society and show off, and are not put down. This is because they made their money outside and that doesn't threaten the resources of the group. The emphasis on that kind of obstacle to change is that of an anthropologist looking at the society as it is without recognizing the possibilities for change as a result of outside influences.

You also talked about organizations rather as if one has to accept the existence of organizations, bureaucracies and hierarchies as they are, and then see how they work. Surely one has to ask under what situations hierarchical authority is necessary? There are basically three ways for coordinating people's economic behaviour in order to ensure production: one is by everybody being motivated to produce something individually which he will sell for money or exchange for some other value with other people (the value may be prestige or status, in certain circumstances); so the producer is motivated without being directed by anybody or agreeing with anybody about what he shall do; if you like, the market situation. The second is the hierarchical authority structure in which someone at one level tells others at a lower level what they should do, and that is necessary for getting certain things done.

There is a third level, that of cooperative decision-making whereby everybody knows the ends of the whole effort; they all take part in the decision about what those ends should be and how each person should contribute to their realization. Then they are motivated to do their best directly for the organization's ends, not because they are paid to do a little bit towards it. To some extent, we are already used to this situation as professionals, although in a capitalist society there is always at the same time the fact that we are motivated to become professionals, and to join our particular organizations, by the salaries we receive (and it is the same in that other society of hierarchical authority structures, the Soviet Union); it can therefore only be to a limited extent, in our work within our organizations, that we are directly motivated by the ends of the organization. You have to see what forms of coordination are most appropriate for the ends you wish to fulfil, rather than look at the ones that exist and point out examples of how they work.

Phoon: It is important, whatever our different perspectives, to understand anthropological and cultural differences, and coming from a multiracial society like Singapore, I think that some of the differences and some of the mental problems and anguish due to industrial growth arise because people do not understand each other and cannot work as a team. We have the indigenous races, also immigrants from Malaysia, and people from the West. They have to acquire social cohesion. In one year in my professional capacity I came across people from 16 countries—from Africa, Europe, Australia and Ceylon—in Singapore. As an instance, we had an industrial dispute because a Dutchman beckoned to a local person in the wrong way for an Asian person! The man thought the Dutchman was insulting him deliberately. Again in our ships we have to provide sometimes two cooks even for a crew of only ten people because Malays won't eat food cooked by Chinese, because of religious and other differences. In asking people to wear the cartridge form of respirators to protect themselves from toxic fumes, I was surprised to hear a refusal, not because of discomfort, but because it looks like a pig's snout! You have to bear in mind these differences when you try to alleviate the ills of industrial growth.

Papanek: I enjoyed Dr Mars' paper because I think the insights of anthropology are so important, but at the same time, their relevance to the world situation of 1974 should not be misjudged. For example, Dr Mars suggested that in Newfoundland there *was* no large group that could make decisions or accept responsibility. But in some cultures equally without such groups, they can be brought into being quickly. I would point to another historical experience, that of the Navaho Indians who were under pressure of having to make major decisions affecting their future. Suddenly their 'Tribal Council' had to meet, apparently for the first time, in 1938. They said, to the surprise of the anthropologists, 'We'll just have to ask the Council to meet *again*'. [My italics.] The anthropologists working with the Navaho had never heard of a Council and asked when it had last met. After much calculation it was found to have last met 308 years before, since that had been the last time that a tribal council was needed. It has met twice since, incidentally, so there is an increase there!

As a second point, I think that whereas much anthropology was originally descriptive, it has lately become manipulative, often through improper tools—for example, the use of out-of-date dictionaries.

Finally, it is possible to almost play a status game by ascribing certain values to certain populations, anthropologically speaking; thus if you wish to speak for creativity you point to Eskimos as, in my opinion, the most creative people in the world. On the other hand it is possible to point to a South American tribe in which *any* innovation is feared and distrusted. It becomes, especially now, very dangerous to take tribal experiences from here or there and to generalize about a society which is becoming more and more homogeneous. What has disturbed me in our discussions, especially of my own paper, is that we take the one-sided attitude that we are now moving towards the village level, which I believe in very strongly, but we forget that two complementary drives are going on at the same time. One must deal with the village level, but also with the global level. It is impossible to sit in Gary, Indiana, and want the place to be unpolluted, on a village level, because to achieve that you have to talk to people in Chicago, because that is where the wind comes from. We must take a holistic view and look at both sides and see how they complement one another.

Porter: I did not get the impression that Dr Mars was saying more than that if a society wishes to innovate or if a government wants to help a community, it is important to understand how that community operates before you introduce innovation. The role of the anthropologist here seems to be important in helping us to do this. Whether the tools available—for example, the participant interview approach—are the most effective may be a separate question. An example here is the question of control over livestock numbers, which is particularly important in many parts of the world, especially drought-prone marginal pasture areas. The first response to a drought is that people ask you to drill wells to provide water for cattle, and the naive and normal response is to agree. We have spent money in drilling wells in response to such requests; but deserts can be created as a result. With a constant supply of water, people are able to keep more cattle, and the cattle outgrow the available grazing. The whole ecology can thus be destroyed. It is then argued that if a constant water supply is to be provided by drilling wells there must be control over grazing; but unless the nature of the society which owns the cattle is thoroughly understood, this is extremely difficult to do. What Dr Mars was discussing can be exemplified by the question of how you engage the population to identify collectively an interest in limiting livestock numbers, when the individual interest of each person is to have as many cattle as possible. This is not a simple problem and it requires much study. I have myself become increasingly sceptical of the value of 'expatriate' anthropologists; the real advance in this direction will come when the developing countries have their own anthropologists to help them to understand the nature of their own societies which they themselves are trying to change, and must change. This makes one more aware of the limitations of what can be done from outside the system. It has to be done from within, because development processes are more difficult and complicated than we ever thought.

Mars: I am afraid I cannot accept Dr White's strictures on the role of anthropologists and their alleged involvement in serving various establishments; that is, colonialism at an earlier period and those whom he now sees acting as proponents of industrialization. The vast majority of anthropologists both today and before Malinowski's time—before the 1920's—have not actively attempted to influence, change or to 'represent' the people they studied or to help the rulers. They have for the most part merely been concerned to examine and record how indigenous cultures operate, motivated to this end simply by a spirit of scientific enquiry. They have been quite grateful that in the vast majority of cases their findings have in fact been ignored by ruling administrations. Indeed, when not ignored, the anthropologist has often found himself criticized or refused access by administrations because they, like he, sometimes appear to distrust the idea that research in these fields can be carried out without some ulterior—that is, usually, a political—involvement.

The point raised about equilibrium traps is well taken. It is certainly true that if peasants move out of their society, become rich and then return, they are likely to spearhead change on their return. I would also agree that one has to ask under what situations hierarchical authority is necessary, though I might prefer to waive the value judgement involved in assessing 'necessities' of this order. But my point was that innovative health care often involves a specific approach at a specific time which must take the society as it is. And when I was talking about hierarchical authorities, I was not concerned with the indigenous hierarchies, vital though their role is in innovation and which, again in the short term, must be regarded as a given, but with the cultures and the dynamics within innovating bureaucracies themselves, which can, one hopes, be amended more easily. The real point is that I am not so much concerned with 'ways of coordinating people's economic behaviour in order to ensure production', as Dr White puts it, but rather in ways of coordinating cooperation and consultation in order to innovate health care.

Dr Papanek's points are, I think, very useful, particularly on the necessity of taking a widely holistic view—of considering that the wind in Gary *does* come from Chicago or, as Mr Porter's example showed, that governments cannot just consider a culture in say Chad, according only to its members' own definitions of their individual situations. This means that the applied anthropologist's role is of necessity very different from that of the usual isolated micro-researcher and here he can face the ethical problem of his relationship to the establishment. As Mair[9] and others have put it, 'you do not tell people what to do so much as what to know'. He is a resource that must increasingly work as one member of a coordinated interdisciplinary team whose problems of coordination are themselves considerable and who can, in their collectivity, only offer solutions as advisers to what he hopes are wise governments. If he considers their motives malevolent he will, I would hope, withdraw. As I see it, his role is to get cognizance taken of the views and interests of the people involved and to do this as they perceive them themselves. If he can open up channels for ongoing consultative involvement that exist after he has gone, so much the better.

References

1. FOSTER, G. M. (1965) *Traditional Cultures and the Impact of Technological Change*, Harper & Row, New York
2. MARRIOTT, McKIM (1955) Western medicine in a village of northern India. In *Health, Culture and Community* (Paul, B. D., ed.), pp. 239-268, Russell Sage Foundation, New York

3. FOSTER, G. M. (1969) *Applied Anthropology*, chapter 3, Little, Brown, Boston
4. BUTCHER, D. (1965) Social survey. In *Volta Resettlement Symposium Papers*, Volta River Authority, Accra
5. KALITSI, E. A. K. (1965) Organization and economics of resettlement. In *Volta Resettlement Symposium Papers*, Volta River Authority, Accra
6. BRIDGER, H., MARS, G., MILLER, E., SCOTT, S. & TOWELL, D. (1973) *An Exploratory Study of the Rcn Membership*, Royal College of Nursing, London
7. BRIDGER, H. (1972) Course designs and methods within the organization. In *Group Training Techniques* (Berger, E. D. S. M. & P., eds.), pp. 34-47 (see particularly p. 41), Gower Press, London
8. FRANKENBERG, R. & LEESON, J. (1974) In *Sociology and Development* (de Kadt, E. & Williams, G., eds.), Tavistock Publications, London
9. MAIR, L. (1969) *Anthropology and Social Change* (London School of Economics Monographs), p. 16, Athlone Press, London

General discussion

Ashby: At the end of a symposium of this kind we need to consider how the good ideas that have come up in our discussion could be turned into action. If we are to try to do this we have first to grapple with the word 'politics' that so far has almost been left out. I don't mean party politics: I mean political systems. I think we agree that there is great scope and need for improvement in the health and sanitary services everywhere, including the developed countries. We agree also that industrial growth has great benefits; and we are not here to discuss zero-growth, or the retreat, as some utopians are urging, to a Rousseau-esque village life, even though many of us see virtue in the organization of societies into small units. There are three questions about possible solutions that should be asked, or three categories of solution, and it may help to try to put our proposed solutions into one of the three categories:

1. Can the changes be made within the present political system of your country?
2. If not, can they be made provided there are *constitutional* changes in the political system of your country? Here I do not exclude the emergence of a different pattern of government (even a Communist government would not be constitutionally impossible in the UK; the Communist Party is not illegal here. So that would be a constitutional change).
3. If neither of those two is true, are the suggestions practicable only provided there is a complete overthrow of the political system of your country? It is, of course, a view shared by some reformers that until you have a revolution, you are wasting your time talking about these other issues. It would help to clarify our thinking if we could decide that what we want done could not be done without a revolution, or calls only for a different pattern of government established by constitutional means, or

needs no more than administrative changes within existing patterns of government.

I was tempted, until I talked with Ivan Illich recently, to add a fourth category—namely, can change be made without changing human nature? Perhaps it isn't fair on him or on ourselves to suggest that as an alternative!

Kirov: Since we are agreed that industrial growth in itself is beneficial, can we add a further question to those posed by Lord Ashby, namely, can this industrial growth be sustained on a world scale within the limited natural resources that we have, and the growing pressure of populations, with the world population expected to double in the next 30 years?

Lawther: It might be useful if this symposium were to come out with a plea for what I consider to be a vital need—that there be a rigorous assessment of the criteria, the guidelines, the standards, now being imposed on many countries that are becoming industrialized, to an extent which is producing economic distress out of all proportion to the good they purport to do. I have seen standards adopted by which a factory could not be built if air pollution were to exceed an annual average of 0.01 p.p.m. of sulphur dioxide—a meaningless figure clinically, but it has closed factories. I have seen test criteria developed on 'scientific' methods which if I hadn't seen them myself I would not have believed. I have also seen the diesel vehicle, one of the most economic forms of transport, banned from at least one country because its exhaust contains 3,4-benzpyrene. Diesel smoke can contain polycyclic hydrocarbons but there is no evidence that they are harmful in these concentrations. We get applications to assess grants from developing countries to have costly spectrophotometers to study polycyclic aromatic hydrocarbons when really they need a mass miniature radiological service. In one country I have seen the application of erroneous blood carbon monoxide measurements which led to policemen having gas masks and oxygen cylinders, because nobody looked critically enough at the results of the analytical methods used. I have seen samples taken for sophisticated measurements to be made by complex and costly apparatus, but the 'sharp end'—the sampling head—has been a cocoa tin lid, which permitted the escape of over 90% of the material sampled.

There is also a great need for a stringent revision of the standards of editing scientific publications in this field. Some of the papers being published, some of which are forming the bases of laws, have clearly never been refereed. One paper, on which a law has been based, stated that 23% saturation by carbon monoxide was produced in a subject inhaling 100 parts per million of the gas. In fact you cannot, even if you inhale carbon monoxide at 100 p.p.m. to infinity, go beyond about 13.4%. Some standards, based on dubious work, are

being applied at huge cost, revolutionizing or imposing great strain on industries and on economies, without there having been any critical examination
of the data. We would do well to say that the concern with some of the
evils of increasing industrialization has led to a slap-happy and slack evaluation
of the data.

Ashby: One ought to be looking to United Nations agencies for international
standards about these things. Internationally agreed methods of analysis are
needed.

Lawther: We have prepared the WHO monograph on the standard methods
for determining many of these values, in each case tailoring the methods
appropriately to the needs of developed and developing countries, not saying
that you need a mass spectrograph if you are going to do it in a poor country.
There have been sad episodes where, even under the aegis of WHO, had I not
protested, some would have set up a network of stations to measure sulphur
dioxide from the combustion of oil, to investigate the possible cause of asthma,
when in fact there was no sulphur in the oil being considered. This kind of thing
is spreading much alarm. In the Gravely Hill case in the UK, in which attempts
are being made to assess the significance of lead pollution, the poverty and
variability of techniques has proved very serious, and has made the results of
the survey very difficult to interpret. I want to make a plea for better science
here.

Ashby: And this is happening in sophisticated as well as unsophisticated
countries; for example the US tried to ban phosphates from detergents (on the
grounds that they destroy the biosphere of lakes) not only in States where there
are great lakes, but in States where there are no lakes at all!

Philip: Maurice Strong and the UN Environment Programme are, doubtless,
doing their best; but I feel I must sympathize with Dr Lawther's jeremiad.
There simply is not the basic information (or, I fear, the basic understanding)
to enable definitive decisions to be made on priorities, standards, and guidelines
for monitoring the whole gamut of recognized environmental pollutants. So
far as UNEP is concerned, I was saddened, though not surprised, to learn that
some provisional priorities and standards were settled recently through the
process of a committee of 'experts' taking votes!

El Batawi: I am very grateful for what Professor Lawther has said and I
agree with him. I have witnessed a meeting of consultants where rather
dogmatic statements were made about the possible health effects of exposure
to different concentrations of pollutants. Although community air pollution
has resulted in episodes of mortality like the London smog, there has been
little evidence of harmful effects on health from general pollutants at prevailing
concentration levels in most countries. Pollution may aggravate chronic

bronchitis and may be associated with other conditions, but the whole thing is felt by many people to be exaggerated. The Human Environment Conference of the UN, in my own personal opinion (which may not be that of WHO) did less good than was hoped for; it emphasized the 'environment' but not as much the human being. It was not very easy to communicate to that conference the health aspects and only about half the governments represented had sent health people.

Exposure to pollution inside industrial enterprises is usually high, resulting, particularly in developing countries, in actual cases of poisoning and permanent disability. With a new emphasis on general pollution, these were given relatively lower priority by some institutions for some time. The environment took the attention and when the appeal came up to ban DDT, the birds in Sweden were more important than human beings in India, who are suffering from a shortage of DDT and the spread of malaria. For all these reasons, we should not exaggerate, and we should evaluate the real effects and not pass judgement without real knowledge that a certain environmental exposure results in ill-health.

With respect to the occupational environment, we know that in many industrialized countries where physical and chemical exposures have been successfully controlled, many of the occupational diseases have disappeared. But occupational diseases dating back to early in the western Industrial Revolution are now appearing in developing countries, but in a different pattern. They are aggravated by communicable diseases, by a bad liver, by low blood haemoglobin, and by many other factors prevailing in the community. They are also aggravated by combined exposures to different stresses outside and inside work. With respect to standards, we have a dilemma in that in some Eastern European countries the permissible levels of toxic agents are generally lower than in the US and western countries. It is usually difficult to reach agreement on these standards, perhaps because of differences in scientific approach or other factors. We cannot affect the political factors, but at least we can approach the technical aspects, and we can organize meetings on comparisons of the methods used, say, in the USSR and US, in establishing biologically safe limits of toxic substances; we may find areas of agreement. We would be happy to see an area of common ground. I believe one of the major responsibilities of WHO is to find those areas of agreement and let each country decide for itself the point on the curve of dose–response relations which will be considered 'safe', allowing for practicability, feasibility, degree of ill-health, effects of combined exposure, and so on.

The vinyl chloride episode with liver cancer has resulted in much publicity in the US because of a few fatal cases. But how many people have died of fibrotic lung disease in the same period, which has been known for years? How many people died in the same period from accidents at work, which are preventable? Why didn't these reach the headlines, as the vinyl chloride episode has done? We should always be level-minded about priorities in research and disease control. Going back to Lord Ashby's questions, I have lived in many countries and have seen different political systems and structures. I don't think we need what he called the third alternative of revolution, in order to introduce change, even in some difficult social structures.

As an example where a political decision is required, take the integration of all the services dealing with the health of working populations. Suppose that we want to move the factory inspectorate of health and safety from the Department of Employment in the UK to the Department of Health, and make the latter responsible for workers' health as a part of the health of the community. If you go between officials at the level of the chief inspector of factories or the head of health services, they will probably not agree with each other because they are in competitive posts. At the level of Ministers, they are also in competitive posts, but if you go up to the top authority, the people who are making the laws, within the constitutional structure of the country, that is where a decision of this kind *can* be taken.

Ashby: So your answer is that solutions must lie in the first category!

Sakabe: Threshold Limit Values (TLV) or standards in the work environment have been settled by specialists in this field, but I wonder whether the TLV can be determined by industrial health specialists alone, or not. The British Occupational Hygiene Society recommended 2 fibres/cm^3 as the standard for chrysotile asbestos dust. The philosophy behind this recommendation is that the risk of developing early clinical signs will be less than 1 % for 50 years' exposure in a working environment containing 2 fibres/cm^3 of chrysotile asbestos dust. This means that 100 workers among 10 000 workers may suffer from early signs of asbestosis for 50 years' exposure. As far as asbestosis is concerned, this decision seems reasonable because the early signs of asbestosis have no serious effect on workers' health. However, in the field of occupational cancer, the situation is very serious.

The philosophy of 'no TLV' seems scientific, but this means theoretically the banning of all carcinogenic substances. We have recognized empirically that there is a difference in carcinogenic potency among these substances. When such substances have rather weak potency and are valuable and useful in people's lives, we are compelled to settle on a TLV or standard for these substances. In such a case, nobody can guarantee that the chosen TLV is completely safe. An important question is: who is responsible for the death from an occupational cancer which might occur in a working environment which would satisfy the TLV? Here, the concept of a socially acceptable level or guarantee of level seems to be useful. Accordingly, the TLV's of occupational carcinogenic substances would be better considered from the standpoints of workers, employers, and government.

Gilson: One may reach agreement on the biological aspects of the dose-response relationship of a toxic substance, but the final Threshold Limit Values are not based solely on the biological evidence but also on the social, economic, and other factors in a particular country. There is a danger of setting universal international standards. It may be better to provide suggested target figures for incorporating in codes of practice, which can be modified to suit the economic and other factors in a particular country at a particular time. It is important to emphasize this because there is an increasing bureaucracy trying to set standards which will supposedly be better because they are international. Another aspect of this problem of setting standards is the lack of good information on the *relative* risks of diseases related to occupation and those, for example, caused by infectious diseases or a range of chronic diseases. It is difficult even in the UK to find good figures of the mortalities associated with different occupations, but what we do have show rather remarkable consistency, and to some extent the same is true between countries; for example, there are enormous differences, of more than a hundred-fold, between occupational fatal accidents in the clothing and in the trawler industries[1]. We need to stimulate the collection of better comparative information of this kind, because it is needed by those making decisions on where to put effort most effectively into reducing occupational hazards.

Dickinson: To return to Professor Lawther's comments, might I say that some of his remarks seem to be a rather slapstick approach to what goes on in some developing countries! The way people gain experience is really the crux of what he is talking about. How do people in these countries make value judgements, about industrialization and industrial problems, in the absence of the wide range of experience that we have had since the Industrial Revolution, with the Alkali Inspectorate and all the rest to collect and collate such experience? We must try to help them become self-critical and learn from their own mistakes, which, inevitably, will be many, as we know from our own experience of all kinds of institutions and activities. We should do all we can to accelerate their experience by providing the best standards from our own experience, but these must be offered for consideration rather than be dictated by WHO or anyone else. Development means gaining experience, learning from mistakes, practising value judgements and gaining self-confidence as much as it means increasing the supply of goods. In the last resort we have to recognize that if something goes *right*, in a development situation, that is good luck. You learn only by analysing the things that go wrong.

Lawther: This wasn't what I meant! I was not criticizing the standards in developing countries; I was criticizing the standards which the developed countries are offering to the developing countries.

White: We must relate the question of standards to the fact that it is in the interests of élites in developing countries to pursue so-called 'higher' standards than are appropriate. These standards are not really better, in many cases, even for them, but they certainly seem higher and more desirable, if only because they are more expensive and more 'modern'. The inappropriate stringency of some environmental pollution standards is related to the inappropriate type or 'standard' of training that doctors and other professionals receive in universities which adopt the curricula of the prestigious institutions of the advanced countries. To take the medical example, doctors are trained to the 'highest' possible standards in most developing countries—partly because in general the educated and the wealthy want what they see as the best medical treatment, and partly because people lucky enough to get medical training want to go on to specialize in order to have a high standard of living, and to be among the élite themselves.

If one looks at what standards are *appropriate*, it might be better to say, for instance, 'Here we have a country of ten million people, with only a few doctors; how best can we care for most of these people?' Let us say that one medical worker can only care for 500–800 people effectively; the appropriate thing to do is to provide, within the resources available, that level of training which will enable us to create ten million divided by 500 or 800 medical workers: that is, 12 500 to 20 000 medical workers (not 'doctors'). That would certainly be in a sense a 'lower' standard of training than if you imposed a standard anything near to that of the western university faculties of medicine (they would know less about a lot of the medicine in the textbooks), but it is the *first* appropriate standard to aim at, and it might well be that they nevertheless had more of the relevant knowledge, and also more empathy with and more willingness to serve the people under their care. I suggest that it would be most appropriate to take people from the local communities, who are motivated to help the community to improve its health by attacking the causes of disease and by applying the treatments they have been taught.

The same thing applies in other fields. Housing is another example: it is often said that 'we must provide a decent standard of housing for the population', particularly in cities of the Third World; but a 'decent' standard of housing within the financial resources of the country means only a few houses being built and often means that other people are cleared off the land in order to build those houses. One finds statements such as 'the road to the airport is lined with slums and we have to make our country beautiful, especially to the foreign tourists who come in from the airport'. And so the slums are pulled down. It is in the interests of the élite that foreign visitors think well of their country. But if you clear people from those slum areas, thousands are deprived of their own solution to their problem, which is the best solution open to them. This is obviously true if you provide no alternative and, very often, indeed none is provided; but it may even be true if you provide a replacement house which seems to *you* better, but do not allow people a free choice between the two (it is likely to be true if you charge a higher rent for the replacement house, or build it further away from opportunities for casual work). So, if we think for the moment just about what can be done within the existing social structure, the first thing we should insist upon is that planners must not prohibit people from doing things unless an alternative is provided for the useful functions that their activity has been performing for themselves or for the community. Planners must provide alternatives that will benefit all the people rather than lay down stringent or 'high' standards which it is only possible to apply to a small minority, who will be raised up into the minute middle-class sitting above the rest of the population.

Dickinson: To take up Professor Kirov's point, I think I am nearer to the 'Doomsday' position than are many others here. I believe that there are non-recurrent raw materials and resources which are finite, and if you are considering that the poorer peoples of the world are to get anything like western standards of living, they are critically finite; so the 'Doomsday' situation is here. There are two things that we must do if we wish to deal responsibly with this situation. As yet we can't, politically or otherwise, accept negative growth, but, as a first step, we must reduce our own energy demands by minimizing energy requirements for processing, manufacturing, and everything else we do; we have to achieve a very strict energy economy. At the same time we have to move over to the use of recurrent resources as fast as possible, and to use the existing critical stock of fossil fuels, in particular, as the capital that will enable us to make this change to a recurrent energy balance society. As people who have used world resources to achieve our high standards of life, we have a duty to everyone in the world to provide the means to achieve adequate, if lower, standards, by adopting a different resource pattern from the one we grew up on. It was a very wasteful pattern and the result was polluting, partly because we wasted instead of using the by-products as raw materials for other processes; we didn't consume our own smoke—in many senses. This gives us the obligation to use our vast resource of professional skills to develop low-energy technology based on recurrent energy resources for our own survival as well as to meet the requirements of those who will never have access to the range of resources we used to consider essential.

Philip: Mr Dickinson has entered a qualification to Lord Ashby's statement that we all agree that industrial growth is a good thing (like the flag, mother, and apple pie), and I join him in this qualification. Some of us certainly don't believe that the existing pattern of industrial growth, if continued, is at all acceptable.

Ashby: I was making the point that we have no right to deprive countries which haven't yet had any industrial growth of the opportunities of having *some*, merely because we have too much.

Philip: One must, of course, agree with that; but it does not seem to be the essential point at issue. Dickinson's point (I think, and certainly mine) is that industrial growth for its own sake is not necessarily desirable: least of all if it takes the form of blind imitation of the course of industrial growth in the developed countries. Surely we must hope that the developing countries will learn from our mistakes. It is true that this is probably a vain hope until the developed countries themselves are seen to have learnt something.

Jones: Surely, because resources are finite, we must try to order the disposition of resources, both material and people, against a series of agreed priorities in the health field. These interactions are inextricably associated with industrial growth. For example, does a country really need a national airline, when it lacks sufficient fertilizer plants?

Papanek: While I share this concern for the depletion of resources, I cannot see people sitting in a room in London making decisions about whether some other country needs a national airline, or an atomic reactor, or first-grade or second-grade roads. In each case it is for that country to decide and it is arrogant to assume that people in developing countries don't have the wisdom and intelligence to learn from our mistakes as well as from their own. The point of hope in the situation is that people in developing countries have so *many* of our mistakes to learn from that the duration of their mistake-phase will be much shorter!

To illustrate that with a story: I like eating fresh fish. I have been in fishing villages in Norway in the past two years unable to buy anything except frozen fish imported from elsewhere in Norway, from Japan, or from anywhere in the world. People there have said with evident pride that 'We Norwegians no longer have to eat fish; we can eat steak now'! My point is that now the Norwegians have achieved a 'steak' culture, it will be short-lived, because in addition to eating steak they also read, and they read that the governments of West Germany, Sweden, the US and many other technologically advanced countries are spending vast sums trying to get people to eat less steak, because they don't enjoy the spectacle of their best managerial talent dying of a coronary thrombosis at the age of 40 or 38. So, there will be a rather short-lived steak culture in Norway, much shorter-lived than in the US or Germany or Japan. That is the one hope for the future, that the phase of industrialization, which in my opinion all countries will be going through that have not gone through it yet, will be on a smaller and more human and briefer scale.

Challis: A theme that has emerged in this symposium has been the need for the underdeveloped countries to produce their own effective organizational structures for dealing with population problems. In this conference the problem has been health. In another it might have been law and order, or industrial worker safety, or whatever. I believe that the conference displays very clearly the problems of a professional class in spreading its valuable expertise widely in an uneducated population—problems of rejection of the advice, but also problems of resistance within the profession towards the reduced élitism which spreading that advice demands.

This leads me to a point that has perhaps been implicit rather than explicit: the need for humility amongst the professional classes if their abilities are to benefit mankind widely. This is particularly true for the less developed countries where emotional and irrational resistance to change is more present (I judge) than in countries with better education and better communications.

Humility is an old-fashioned word, and there will be better jargon words to dress up the concept. But with humility comes integrity and the ability to *listen* to others. I am sure that the fierce battles of experts in the conferences of international organizations are as symptomatic of lack of humility as are the problems of recognizing the 'barefoot doctor'. Perhaps the Chinese have a basic humility!

Illich: Lord Ashby has proposed that we translate the dynamics of industrial health hazards into terms that can be discussed as political issues. I welcome this proposal, as long as we are willing to face two correlated challenges. On the one hand, we ought to look at dose–response relationships not only in technical but also in social terms; on the other, we ought to formulate overall negative design characteristics for industrial processes in political terms which do not require professional intervention in order to be turned into legal provisions.

So far we have looked at the dose–response relationship as if tolerable nuisance could be reduced to the organic response to merely material impacts. We have explored the existence of tolerable thresholds to physical stress. Analogous thresholds exist also in a social and psychological dimension. Only within these thresholds does the organism remain capable of coping with its environment in an autonomous way. When the physical or the social environment is distorted beyond certain thresholds, the organism remains viable only if it is increasingly serviced, maintained and managed in a heteronomous way. Coping degenerates into maintenance, with or without consent of the maintained.

Let me illustrate this. As machines are speeded up, increasingly protective gear is needed to safeguard the worker. As increasingly toxic substances enter into the production process, increasingly costly defensive devices will have to shield the worker and the consumer from their material impact. Both of these are costly buffers necessary to keep the response to doses of industrial environmental change within the limits tolerable to human beings.

With the very same degree of necessity with which industrial efficiency renders the process faster and more poisonous, it also renders it more complex, more standardized and more opaque. People cease to be able to grasp, to respond, and to feel on their own. At this point the industrial system would break down if a kind of immaterial buffer were not provided by tertiary economic activities. This buffer takes the form of education, personnel administration and medical care.

We must see material and immaterial buffers as two industrially created demands of the same kind. In comparison with the former, the latter are enormously more costly, more alienating, and more destructive of the worker's autonomy. People have only a limited capacity to undergo pedagogical, bureaucratic or medical therapies before their health breaks down.

This statement is based on a certain view of health. As I understand the issue, health is an ordinary word which designates the level of autonomy with which an organism is capable of coping with its environment. As long as this relationship remains a non-trivial one for the organism, we say that it is healthy. When the organism needs to consume more and more products put out by some service industry, the autonomy of its relationship to the environment declines and its health—by definition—decreases. In other words, medical care given to keep people on an inhuman job must come to a point at which these services have health-denying effects.

The second matter is related to this. Who shall determine at what point the volume of effective medical interventions at the service of an industrial society begins to engender health-denying effects? Who shall decide at which point technically effective industrial hygiene and medicine begin to engender iatrogenic effects of a more general kind? Who shall determine the thresholds not only of the material and non-material dose of impact which workers can tolerate, but also (and that is the critical issue here) the levels of institutional (and therefore heteronomous) assistance they shall be obliged to accept in order to be enabled to stay on the job?

If the power to define what is tolerable were transferred to experts, one basic aspect of human health would be expropriated. Consciously to face the challenge of the environment or to attempt withdrawal is a basic attribute of human autonomy, which constitutes health. In order for the limitation of industrial impact to be achieved, and also the limitation of tolerable management of the response to remain 'healthy', they must be the outcome of conscious and non-trivial initiatives of the people who are affected by the decision. For general reasons of health, limits to the industrial outputs of material and immaterial products must be set in a political process. Experts might help to clarify issues and options; that is as far as they can go.

Kissick: This symposium has been an extraordinary experience for me. We have discussed Health and Industrial Growth, both of which I once thought were absolute concepts. Both, I am now convinced, are relative ones, and both, even health, are means to an end. The World Health Organization notwithstanding, health alone, I suspect, is not enough. There has to be a purpose beyond it for which man can use his health. Industrial growth is also a means to an end—that is, to achieving things as basic as food and shelter, and things as esoteric, but probably over-riding, as civilization.

My perspective is predominantly that of a former Director of Program Planning and Evaluation, in the Office of the Surgeon General (US Public Health Service), responsible for trying to formulate investment decisions vis-à-vis a few thousand million dollars to influence a rather complex social institution—the health care enterprise. We in the US, contrary to world opinion, are a federation of developed and underdeveloped communities. We appear extraordinarily affluent, which we are; but we also contain extraordinary deficiencies. By the end of 1975, our health enterprise will probably exceed a hundred thousand million American dollars, or approximately £40 000 million sterling. That will represent 8–9% of our Gross National Product; the percentage, of course, will be determined by the growth rate for GNP, which is now slowing down. In the midst of all this, the United States as a society is beginning to recognize that it can't do everything it wants to at one and the same time. Throughout our history, we have had the pleasure of buying our way out of our problems; now we have to plan and choose. This is very difficult.

So, where are we? To return to health, I think we should be guided by a paraphrase of Clemenceau: health is too important to be left to physicians. Almost a decade has passed since I first published that statement; I now would amend it to include all health professionals. What we have to offer was suggested by several members of this symposium, but probably most focally in our consideration of anthropology. As professionals we need to learn how to become consultant collaborators rather than the professionals who dictate solutions. We should rather ask, can I help formulate a solution by examining the alternatives? Because Health and Industrial Growth are relative, we are talking about choices, risks, values or alternatives. We professionals can help. We have the technology to help; data, computers, simulations, and so on, enable us to suggest certain choices with specific implications in so many years. Let us reflect on these opportunities.

Where do I come out? With the soft sciences, not the hard sciences. Our problems are more those of political economy than they are of precise measurement of physical parameters in the environment.

It is significant that we are discussing these issues within the homeland of Adam Smith, Malthus and John Maynard Keynes. What the developed world—western societies—is groping for now is some 'Post-Keynsian' theory of political economy that will enable us to collaborate, help, share, respond, grow, and survive. So to a question, which leaves me ending where Lord Ashby began—Cardinal Newman's statement: 'Many a man will live and die upon a dogma: no man will be a martyr for a conclusion'. Can our conclusion become a dogma? I wonder whether that tortured intellect who spent so many years in the British Museum formulating a conclusion did not indeed come forth with a dogma.

From this symposium, I take away what I call the Carlsberg phenomenon: the realization that a free-enterprise, corporate endeavour, which I assume is profit-seeking, can rise above principle to solve an industrial problem. I do indeed want to find out more of the specifics: it is a bias of mine that the irrationality of man is frequently more creative than destructive, and frequently leads to civilization rather than entropy. If somebody asked me for a proposal, I would suggest that rather than 'world socialism', as has been proposed here, we think about world heterodoxy—that is, a radical heterodoxy—with radical convictions, radical conceptualizations, radical enquiry, radical techniques and, beyond this, radical implementation. Lacking alternatives, we shall prove capable!

References

1. POCHIN, E. E. (1974) Occupational and other fatality rates. *Community Health* 6, 2-13

Conclusions

ERIC ASHBY

If we had been discussing some narrow theme in medical science we could, at this stage, sum up the 'state of play' in the subject, separating out what is known, what is still conjecture, and what the next steps in advance are likely to be. Our theme is far too broad for such a simple summary. Indeed, if one thing stands out more clearly than anything else from our discussions, it is the unpredictable *interdependence* of health, industrial growth, and the patterns of society in the countries from which we come, and the complexity of the network of relationships between them. How could any planner have foreseen the effect of industrial growth on farmers in Iran, or the Volta dam on fishermen in Ghana? (Or, to come nearer home, will planners foresee the effects of North Sea oil on Scottish crofters? I doubt it.) Some of the political and social problems which arise as second-order effects of industrialization do not seem susceptible to rational analysis at all. And even when there are rational solutions to problems they are not (as solutions to scientific problems are) valid everywhere. Each society has to solve its own social problems in its own style.

What, then, has been the value of these three days of discussion among people from nine different countries? I think we have discovered that every country represented here has something to learn from other countries and something to teach to other countries.

Let me select a few of these lessons. One is that the 'common man' should not, in health (or in anything else, for that matter), become parasitic upon experts. Health education should equip people to take some responsibility for their own health. A second lesson is that administrative fragmentation can be inimical to health services, for instance by separating responsibility for a man's health in the factory from his health (and that of his family) at home; or by separating responsibility for the planning of new industries or new factories

251

from responsibility for the sanitation and living conditions of the surrounding community. A third lesson (learnt at great cost by some impoverished countries which have imported, without change, medical systems from affluent countries) is that a nation's medical service should be designed to serve the whole of the population, not just a small urbanized élite; even though this calls for the training of a large corps of medical assistants who would not be qualified to practice in highly industrialized countries. A fourth lesson is that industrial growth generates health problems which may not fall within the ambit of conventional medical care: stress due to noise, or pollution, or the demands made by modern machinery—all the disorders lumped together as psychosocial. We were reminded too (a fifth lesson) that the admirable health-and-welfare schemes of big multinational corporations do not cover, even in affluent countries, the 'typical' worker. He is likely to be in a small—perhaps a 'backyard'—factory, without adequate protection against the hazards of his trade.

A sixth lesson is that even the most sophisticated attempts at 'technology assessment' (such as the very thorough studies which preceded the building of the Volta dam) cannot be relied upon to give trustworthy predictions. This is not to say that they are not worth doing: far from it. But we have to resign ourselves to the hard fact that huge social experiments (which is what industrial growth is) have, and will continue to have, surprising and sometimes distressing results. All the more need, therefore, to monitor them (and this is the next lesson), to keep scrupulous records, so that the results of health services can be evaluated. To sum it all up, I like to think of our days of discussion as a mosaic of ideas, which can be put into new and useful combinations in the countries from which we come.

Biographies of contributors

ERIC ASHBY   Born in 1904. His professional career was in experimental botany and he published many papers on the analysis of growth in plants. He was professor first in Sydney and then in Manchester. In 1950 he became President and Vice-Chancellor of the Queen's University of Belfast and in 1959 Master of Clare College, Cambridge. For many years he took part in the planning and development of universities in tropical Africa and he was chairman of the commission which produced a blueprint for higher education in Nigeria. From 1970 to 1973 he was chairman of the Royal Commission on Environmental Pollution in Britain. He is the author of several books on comparative higher education, including *Universities: British, Indian, African* (Weidenfeld & Nicolson 1966), which is a history of the 'export' of universities to these countries over the last century.

M. BAVANDI   Born in 1934 in Iran. He is now the Deputy Director of the Division of Health and Social Welfare in the Plan and Budget Organization. He formerly served as the Research Supervisor at the Food and Nutrition Institute of Iran and as Assistant Dean and Lecturer in the School of Nutritional Sciences.

HAROLD BRIDGER   Is Programme Director, Career Development and Institutional Change, at the Tavistock Institute of Human Relations, of which he was a founder member. Originally a mathematician, he qualified as a psychoanalyst in 1950. He is currently concerned with research and development in group and organizational processes, and cross-cultural and multidisciplinary activities. He is a member of the Area Health Authority for Camden and Islington in London. Relevant papers include, with Miller and O'Dwyer, *The Doctor and Sister in Industry* (Macmillan 1963) and Aspects of Expatriate Family Moves (in *Proceedings of the International Conference on Occupational Health*, 1973).

EDWARD JOHN CHALLIS   Born in London in 1925, and qualified as a chemical engineer in London University in 1946. Currently the Production and Environment Director of Petrochemicals Division of Imperial Chemical Industries Limited. Has been

253

involved in the production of petrochemicals for over 20 years, mostly in the design and operation of continuous automatically controlled process plant. Has worked on research into the application of econometric computer control to such plants, and was responsible for the first such installation in ICI Limited in the early 1960's. Based in the North-East of England where there is a massive group of petrochemical production plant, he has a strong interest in the environmental and human welfare problems which such operations bring to both the workers within the factory and the surrounding community. He has published a number of papers on this theme.

L. K. A. DERBAN   Born in 1928 in Ghana. Is the Chief Medical Officer of the Volta River Authority, Accra, Ghana. From 1966 to 1973 he was on the staff of the Department of Community Health, University of Ghana Medical School. His specialty is occupational health. He is a member of the WHO Expert Panel on Occupational Health. He also serves as a consultant to a number of industries in Ghana on matters of occupational health.

HAROLD DICKINSON   Born in 1924 in Bury, Lancashire, England. At present is at the School of Engineering Science at the University of Edinburgh, where his main interests lie in the fields of energy conversion and the transfer of technologies to poor countries. He has worked in a number of developing countries as consultant, United Nations expert and university teacher.

MOSTAFA A. EL BATAWI   Born in 1928 in Cairo, Egypt. He graduated in Medicine at the University of Cairo in 1951 and subsequently became Fellow and Master of Public Health and Doctor of Science in Occupational Health, at the University of Pittsburgh. From 1960 to 1965 he was Head of the Department of Occupational Health at the University of Alexandria and later Professor of the same department. He was ILO Regional Adviser for Occupational Health in Asia during 1965-1969, and since then has been Chief Medical Officer for the Occupational Health Programme of WHO in Geneva.

JOHN C. GILSON   Born in 1912 near Birmingham, England. Is Director of the Medical Research Council Pneumoconiosis Unit in South Wales. He has been concerned with research into occupational and environmental respiratory diseases, especially those arising in coal-mining, the cotton industry, and workers exposed to asbestos dust. He has been active in promoting international studies of the health hazards of asbestos in association with the International Agency for Research on Cancer at Lyon.

WALTER W. HOLLAND   Born in 1929. Has been Professor of Clinical Epidemiology and Social Medicine at St Thomas's Hospital Medical School since 1968, and Honorary Director of the St Thomas's Social Medicine and Health Service Research Unit. He has been Visiting Professor at Monash University, Melbourne and at the University of California at Los Angeles. He was elected a member of the Johns Hopkins University Society of Scholars in 1970.

IVAN ILLICH   Born in 1926 in Vienna, Austria. Since 1960 he has been an independent student associated with CIDOC in Cuernavaca in Mexico. He was previously Vice-Chancellor in the University of Pouce, Puerto Rico. He is author of *Celebration of Awareness* (1968), *De-Schooling Society* (1970), *Tools for Conviviality* (1972), *Energy and Equity* (1973) and *Medical Nemesis: The Expropriation of Health* (1974) (all published by Calder & Boyars, London).

W. T. JONES   Born 1927 in Maryport, England. Until end of 1974 was Senior Lecturer in Occupational Health at the TUC Centenary Institute of Occupational Health, London School of Hygiene and Tropical Medicine. Before this he was the first Director General of the Health Education Council. He is now a District Community Physician in the London area. Publications have covered health education, the organization of occupational health services and the use of information systems. With Helen Grahame he is co-author of *Health Education in Great Britain* (to be published in 1975).

NIKOLAS Y. KIROV   Born in 1920 in Sofia, Bulgaria. Is Head of the Department of Fuel Technology at the University of New South Wales in Sydney, Australia. He is a consultant of WHO, Western Pacific Region, on combustion technology, incineration and air pollution control. He has also worked in several research organizations and academic institutions in the UK and in North America.

WILLIAM L. KISSICK   Born in 1932 in Detroit, Michigan, USA. Is George S. Pepper Professor of Community Medicine (School of Medicine) and Professor of Health Care Systems (the Wharton School) at the University of Pennsylvania. He previously spent seven years in the Executive Branch of the US Federal Government, responsible for health planning and evaluation, policy formulation and the development of legislative proposals. In 1974-1975 he was Visiting Professor at the University of London and at Leuven University.

P. J. LAWTHER   Born 1921. Educated at Carlisle and Morecambe Grammar Schools, King's College, London, and St Bartholomew's Hospital Medical College. After a year's school-teaching he worked in the chemical industry before reading medicine. After holding clinical and research posts in the Professorial Unit at St Bartholomew's Hospital he joined the Medical Research Council's Scientific Staff in 1954 as Director of the Air Pollution Research Unit. He was formerly Chief Clinical Assistant at the Brompton Hospital, and is now Professor of Environmental Medicine (in the University of London) at St Bartholomew's Hospital Medical College; Physician-in-Charge at the Department of Preventive and Environmental Medicine; and Director of the WHO International Reference Centre on Air Pollution.

GERALD MARS Born in 1933 in Manchester, England. He is currently Nuffield Foundation Social Science Research Fellow and an Associate Consultant of the Tavistock Institute of Human Relations. He has held teaching and research posts in North America and the UK; he lectures at Middlesex Polytechnic at Enfield and has written on industrial sociology, industrial relations and social anthropology. He holds a doctorate in Social Anthropology from the London School of Economics.

ROBERT MURRAY Born in 1916 in Law, Scotland. He was Medical Adviser to the Trades Union Congress until January 1975. He was previously a Medical Inspector of Factories (1947-1956) and a Counsellor in the Occupational Safety and Health Division of the International Labour Office, Geneva (1956-1961). He is the author, with B. H. Harvey, of *Industrial Health Technology* (Butterworths 1958).

VICTOR PAPANEK Born in 1925 in Vienna, Austria. Is a consultant designer for UNESCO, UNIDO, and for 'job enlargement' programmes for corporations in Scandinavian countries. Since leaving his job as Dean of the California Institute of the Arts, he has been working as Visiting Guest Professor in charge of postgraduate industrial design in Denmark (1971-1972) and at Manchester Polytechnic (1973-1975). He spans the disciplines of anthropology and industrial design and has spent several years living with Alaskan, Canadian and Greenland Eskimos, Navaho and Zuni Indians, Lapplanders, and Balinese; and in West and Central Equatorial Africa. He is the author of *Design for the Real World: Human Ecology and Social Change* (1971), *Nomadic Furniture* (with Jim Hennessey, 1973), and *Nomadic Furniture 2* (with Jim Hennessey, 1974) (all published by Pantheon Books, New York). *Design for the Real World* (published in the UK by Thames & Hudson) now exists in 16 languages and in 18 editions and is being translated into seven more languages. Appointed Professor of Industrial Design, Carleton University, Ottawa in 1975.

J. R. PHILIP Born in 1927 in Ballarat, Australia. Is Chief of the CSIRO Division of Environmental Mechanics in Canberra. Over 20 years he has published numerous papers on soil and porous medium physics, fluid mechanics, hydrology, micrometeorology, and mathematical and physical aspects of physiology and ecology. He has held visiting posts at many universities, including Cambridge, California Institute of Technology, and Harvard. He has been involved, at both national and international level, with UNESCO's International Hydrological Decade and Man and Biosphere Programmes. He is Secretary (Biological Sciences) of the Australian Academy of Science and a Fellow of the Royal Society.

WAI-ON PHOON Born in 1932 in Singapore. Since 1970 he has been Professor of Social Medicine and Public Health at the University of Singapore. He was formerly Senior Medical Adviser to Shell Eastern Petroleum Ltd. He is President of the Society of Occupational Medicine in Singapore and a member of the WHO Expert Advisory Committee on Occupational Health. He is Vice-President of the International Association of Traffic and Accident Medicine and a member of the Committee for the Study of Geographical Pathology of the Permanent Commission and International

Association on Occupational Health. He was formerly President of the Singapore Medical Association and was Founder-Chairman of the Singapore Inter-Professional Centre. He has worked as a schoolmaster and held academic posts in bacteriology, paediatrics and internal medicine. He is the author of *Comprehensive Human and Social Biology* (Federal Publications, Singapore 1973) and editor of *Health and Safety at Work* (National Safety First Council, Singapore 1971).

ROBERT S. PORTER   Born in 1924 in London. Is now Director-General of the Economic Planning Staff in the British Ministry of Overseas Development. From 1951 until 1965 he served in the Middle East Development Division, now a regional office of the Ministry of Overseas Development, first in Cairo, then in Beirut, Lebanon. In 1965 he joined the Ministry of Overseas Development as Director of the Geographical Division of the Economic Planning Staff.

V. RAMALINGASWAMI   Born in India in 1921. He is Professor of Pathology and Director of the All-India Institute of Medical Sciences in New Delhi. He is interested in malnutrition and human health and in the education of physicians for developing countries.

H. SAKABE   Born in 1915. Is Chief of the Department of Industrial Physiology at the National Institute of Industrial Health in Kawasaki, Japan. From 1957 to 1967 he served successively as Chief of the Department of Occupational Diseases and Chief of the Department of Industrial Hygiene at the Institute. He has published papers on industrial health and air pollution.

ALASTAIR WHITE   Born in 1941 in London. Now at the Institute of Development Studies, University of Sussex, where he is engaged in a research project on health sector aid to underdeveloped countries. Until recently a lecturer in sociology at the University of Stirling. Has worked on urban sociology in Latin America and on the sociology of development. Author of *El Salvador* (Ernest Benn, London, and Praeger, New York 1973).

JOHN C. WOOD   Born in 1928 at Brighouse, Yorkshire. Is Professor of Law at the University of Sheffield. His main interests are criminal law and industrial law. He was Vice-Chairman of the Robens Committee on Health and Safety at Work (1970-1972).

Index of contributors

Ashby, Lord **3**, 12, 47, 97, 99, 120, 139, 214, 237, 239, 241, 245, **251**

Bavandi, M. **75**, 82, 83, 86
Bridger, H. 25, 27, 66, 98, 149, 153, 155, 193, 200, 210

Challis, E. J. 28, 100, 120, 152, **179**, 193, 194, 213, 246

Derban, L. K. A. **49**, 68, 216
Dickinson, H. 14, 43, 69, 102, 120, 122, 123, 177, 193, 198, 216, 228, 242, 244

El Batawi, M. A. 11, 24, 27, 69, 87, 99, 104, 122, **141**, 154, 167, 195, 216, 229, 239

Gilson, J. C. 27, 100, 196, 242

Holland, W. W. 44, 83, 195

Illich, I. 70, 139, 152, **157**, 166, 168, 216, 229, 246

Jones, W. T. 26, 87, 98, 121, 167, 194, 196, 197, **203**, 245

Kirov, N. Y. **31**, 43, 44, 47, 238
Kissick, W. L. 248

Lawther, P. J. 212, 238, 239, 243

Mars, G. 12, 67, 120, 150, 178, **219**, 229
Murray, R. 124, 197, 212

Papanek, V. 13, 27, 46, 97, 121, **171**, 175, 177, 178, 232, 245
Philip, J. R. 44, 176, 239, 245
Phoon, W. O. 12, **107**, 120, 124, 135, 136, 148, 151, 165, 175, 211, 231
Porter, R. S. 46, 84, 98, 101, 122, 167, 196, 217, 232

Ramalingaswami, V. 14, 47, 82, **89**, 97, 99, 139, 153, 155, 163, 213, 215

Sakabe, H. 100, **127**, 135, 136, 241

White, A. 11, 85, 96, 98, 101, 136, 139, 164, 199, 230, 243
Wood, J. C. **17**, 25, 26, 29

Indexes compiled by William Hill

259

Subject index